INTUITIVE EATING

A REVOLUTIONARY 4-STEP PROGRAM, BASED ON 10
POWERFUL PRINCIPLES, THAT WORKS! HOW THOUSANDS OF
PEOPLE, REWIRING THEIR MINDS, STUCK TO THEIR DIET
AND HAVE LOST MORE THAN 125 POUNDS.

BY MEREDITH CARNEY

TABLE OF CONTENTS

FOREWORD

This integrative function illuminates how reasoning, once regarded as a "purely logical" setting of thinking, is in fact, reliant on the non-rational processing of our anatomies.

Knowing a little about the mind can help to realize why we're born with the wisdom we have to become Intuitive Eaters. Additionally, it may help us to observe how we're in a position to live an Intuitive Consuming life, even while becoming bombarded by the endless options of organic and refined foods open to us every day and the relentless diet plan messages that abound.

Human beings are privileged to see a dynamic interplay of instinct, emotion, and the mind mediates idea, which interacts to orchestrate life, and so. Mindfulness and psychiatrist expert, Daniel Siegel, M.D., calls this technique "Mind-Sight." There are three parts of the brain accountable for this powerful integration.

The first region is named the reptilian brain, since when the first reptiles roamed the planet earth; they acted and responded by instinct exclusively. They didn't rationalize, or feel-they merely went for this. As life evolved, another degree of brain function developed, called the limbic mind, which mammals possess also. Emotions and interpersonal behaviours originate right here. In the human limbic brain, feelings are layered upon the instincts of the reptilian mind. The abilities from the reptilian mind are delivered to the human limbic brain, which serves to increase consciousness. Ultimately, the third key area of the mind evolved, known as the rational mind, or the neo-cortex. The sensible human brain integrates instincts and emotions from the additional two brain regions. The sensible brain will not control instincts-instead; it perceives the instinctual and feeling elements of our beings and displays upon them. The rational mind creates thoughts and vocabulary.

Intuitive Eating embraces most three elements of the human being brain. In toddlerhood and infancy, eating is instinctual mostly. As we get older, thoughts and feelings frequently play a part in our decisions about eating. As we frequently tell our clients, our bodies are not only composed of the tongue and the stomach but the mind also. We've often heard somebody say, "I believed that as an Intuitive Eater, I possibly could eat whatever I needed. So, now I consume whatever I'd like and in so far as I want, whenever I think like it!" In fact, this comment distorts the premise of intuitive feeding. Yes, make peace with meals, and consume what pleases your palate. Yes, provide yourself with the freedom to consume unconditionally, and eat just as much as you need to fulfil the body. But eating once you experience it, without respect for food cravings and fullness may not be an extremely satisfying experience and can even cause physical pain. Attunement, together with your body's satiety cues is usually an important part of the process.

As an Intuitive Eater, you'll be honouring your brain, because it is a component of the body. As you feel the concepts of Intuitive Eating, you'll be storing info in the memory "files" that you produce and house in the human brain. When you are feeling hungry, you will have to pull up a number of these files, while deciding what things to consume. You will evaluate how starving you are feeling and then consider what foods might fulfil your hunger as well as your taste buds. You may actually go through a number of sensual imaginings of the flavour and texture and heat of different foods. You may open the file to reflect on past eating experiences also. You may inquire yourself whether your current eating choice spent some time working out for you personally when you've consumed it previously. Achieved it sustains you very long enough? Achieved it makes your bloodstream sugars crash? Did you finish up with indigestion? Or do you thoroughly benefit from the food and want it again? Your feelings may also come into play when you have the desire to eat. Might you become upset and so are craving foods to comfort and ease and soothe yourself? Or are you bored and considering feeding on as a distraction? Considering these options might inform your decision about what things to eat, or even whether to consume/eat at all.

Initially of your trip to reclaim your Intuitive Eater, you will likely be hyperconscious of hunger, fullness, satisfaction, thoughts, and emotions. The human brain should be extremely in tune together with your tongue as well as your stomach. As you become even more adept at recognizing your internal signals, you might find that your instincts and intuitive wisdom consider even more of a prominent part in your eating encounter. Therefore, Intuitive Eating is actually about trusting you will be capable of accessing all the information you must have, by using all the areas of your brain-your reptilian instincts, your limbic reference to your emotions, as well as your rational thoughts.

Through Intuitive Eating, we figure out how to trust the wisdom which has always been within but has been blunted by years of self-doubt. Doubting their innate consuming signals had prolonged to doubting their beliefs about a great many other areas of their lives.

We've heard stories about individuals who have left abusive associations, made peace with estranged family members, and also have made significant profession changes, once they have a problem with meals and body has been resolved. We have also found out about new romances that, for a few, could not have already been possible while these were occupied with body issues and focused on the most recent doomed diet plan attempt. Intuitive Eating offers freed most of these people to continue with their lives while departing behind self-question and despair.

INTRODUCTION

If you could profit every diet just like a frequent flyer program, the majority of us could have earned a vacation to the moon and back. The almost $60 billion at 12 months, the weight-loss industry could finance the trip for generations to arrive (Bacon and Aphramor 2011). Ironically, we appear to have significantly more respect for our vehicles than for ourselves. If you took your vehicle to a car mechanic for regular tune-ups, and after money and time spent, the automobile didn't function, and you wouldn't blame yourself. Yet, regardless of the fact that 90 to 95 per cent of most diets fail-you have a tendency to blame yourself, not the dietary plan! Isn't it ironic that with an enormous failure price for dieting-we don't blame the procedure of dieting?

Initially, whenever we ventured into the globe of private practice, we didn't know each other. Yet, separately, each folk had remarkably similar guidance experiences that triggered us to rethink how exactly we work. This resulted in a significant change in how exactly we practice and years, later on, was the impetus because of this book.

My objective for Intuitive eating wasn't fame or fortune, however. When I sat right down to write the book, I simply wished to educate and motivate visitors to achieve superior health, whether they wished to lose weight, feel good, or invert a chronic disease. I experienced no idea the publication would take off, or that it could resonate so deeply with people all over the world. It seemed everyone began using that phrase-intuitive eating-to explain the overwhelmingly effective eating design detailed in reserve. And to this full-day, there are apparently never-ending blasts of discussions, describing miraculous health adjustments, caused by this topic.

The trick behind Intuitive eating's popularity is easy: It didn't promise an instant fix. Unlike crash diets that guarantee easy and instant results, "Intuitive eating" organized vital details about food and healthful eating that allowed visitors to be specialists in nutrition. The publication essentially paid to its visitors the keys to effective weight reduction so that these were in charge of their health destiny.

Center to Intuitive eating is a straightforward health equation, the core idea of my nutritarian program:

$H = N / C$ Wellness = Nutrients / Calories

Your wellbeing is predicted by your nutrient intake divided by your calorie consumption.

I contact this core idea the nutrient density of your daily diet. Food gives us nutrition and calorie consumption (energy). All calories result from only three components: carbohydrates, fat, and proteins. Nutrients, however, come from noncaloric food factors, namely, vitamin supplements, nutrients, fibres, and phytochemicals, actually chemical substances that generally occur in plants. These noncaloric nutrients are quite crucial to your wellbeing. When the ratio of nutrition to calorie consumption is high, fat burns up, and wellness is restored. The even more nutrient-dense meals you consume, the, even more, you'll be happy with fewer calories, and the much less you'll crave excess fat and high-calorie foods.

A high-nutrient diet decreases growing older, helps restoration cells, reduces inflammation, and helps rid your body of toxins. High-nutrient, low-calorie foods include a great deal of dietary fibre and take up a whole lot of space in the stomach. As you consume a more substantial quantity of food, it satiates your food cravings and blunts your hunger. Meeting the body's micronutrient requirements also helps suppress food craving and what I contact "toxic hunger, " which drives you to consume more calories than you require-usually in the type of processed foods, which can result in cancer and heart disease, among a great many other ailments.

Witnessing how Intuitive consuming inspired a lot of people to improve their diets not merely reinforced my results that high-nutrient diets create good wellness; it offered a considerable, ongoing body of proof proving that approach works. Nothing displays the energy of this method of consuming more than hearing from individuals who apply this understanding and live it each day in their personal lives. Thousands of individuals lost dramatic levels of weight without problems rather than regained it. One reader called Scott weighed an astounding 500 pounds. Scott couldn't tie his very own sneakers. His breathing was laboured, and he could walk only nine actions at a time. He was thirty-eight years aged. A doctor informed him that if he didn't undergo belly reduction surgery, he'd probably die within half a year. Scott spurned his doctor's guidance and instead made a decision to switch how he considered food and his method of eating by pursuing my high-nutrient meal strategy, which offered him with the nutrients, protein, and vitamin supplements he had a need to achieve good wellness. Because he right now eats for health, he can eat just as much as he wants, ignoring the scale fully. Today, Scott weighs 180 pounds and wants to exercise-a big differ from when he could not walk. My individuals routinely lose up to 20 pounds through the first six weeks of changing their diet plan. And that's simply the start. More importantly, they typically get over diseases such as for example allergies, asthma, acne, headaches, high blood circulation pressure, diabetes, reflux esophagitis, lupus, kidney insufficiency, psoriasis, angina, cardiomyopathy, and multiple sclerosis-and they steadily get to get rid of their dependence on prescription drugs.

Though I have very long studied and utilized high- nutrient eating as a medical prescription for days gone by twenty-five years, actually I must admit to being amazed by a few of the phenomenal recoveries folks have reported if you ask me. Once, somebody asked whether this micronutrient-rich approach could change their hair back again to brownish from grey. "Of program not really," I answered. But, affirmed, on my website discussion board, two different people commented that it experienced occurred to them. I couldn't believe it. Similarly, among my sufferers had hepatitis C prior to starting my eating design. I didn't believe this high-nutrient eating design would remedy his hepatitis contamination and liver injury; nevertheless, after some right time, his hepatitis C disappeared. I had to do it again the blood tests 3 x to believe it. Seeing such dramatic recoveries from what exactly is conventionally considered irreversible illnesses excited me, making me even more adamant that delicious method of eating can result in medical transformations for an incredible number of Americans.

The total results and success stories are astounding. They come from folks of different back again- grounds, from different age groups, and they all began their journeys for different factors. Yet what they talk about in common is all of them are now in excellent wellness. For most of the Intuitive eating's achievement; however, I quickly found realize that science-based details about nutrition only wasn't enough. With these details available to such a wide audience, why would a lot of people neglect to recognize there have to protect their valuable health insurance and lose weight? Why would they become unable and unready to change? Why would they like to reject unassailable, scientific, and significantly effective advice? I'll let you know why, due to the mind-boggling twin powers of meals preference and meals addiction.

Just like the classic victim, we actually grow to love things that kill us-in this case, unhealthy food. Unhealthy eating styles and meals addictions have both used control of our brains, and this dependence on certain foods is frequently as deadly as many other addictions.

The standard American diet plan (SAD) is eliminating us. Rather than providing us with these basic needs once and for all health, it has created a country where disease and persistent illness are believed to be unavoidable and just another organic consequence of ageing. Carrying excess fat is the primary reason behind type 2 diabetes; it accelerates atherosclerosis and death from cardiovascular disease. In just a matter of years, excess body weight is usually projected to overtake smoking as the root cause of loss of life in the USA. By enough time, most Americans reach age fifty, they are already addicted to prescription drugs, and almost fifty per cent of People in America still die of heart attacks and strokes. You don't need to be one of them. Twenty-eight million Americans have problems with the crippling discomfort of osteoarthritis. You do not have to be one of these. Thirty-five million Americans have problems with persistent headaches. You don't need to be one of them. You simply don't need to be sick.

Today, 475 million adults all over the world suffer from obesity. That's a 50 per cent increase since 1980. Simultaneously, the amount of over- excess weight adults is fast approaching 1 billion, plus some 200 million school-age kids are already overweight, which means almost 1. 7 billion individuals are either overweight or obese. One nearly 7 billion people!

In the USA alone, about two-thirds of People in America are overweight, based on the National Institutes of Wellness (NIH). But this doesn't tell the complete story. Both NIH and the Globe Health Business define an "obese" person to possess a body mass index (BMI) of 25. This implies that a woman who is 5 feet 5 inches tall is considered a standard pounds at 150 pounds, and a guy whose 5 feet 10 inches tall is considered regular at 175 pounds. This man and female may carry between 20 and 30 pounds of disease- leading to excess fat around their waists. However, they would be considered healthy and match by today's standards. This is not accurate to look at a person with that very much fat normal or healthy. If you look at societies or groups of individuals who live longer than average, you'll discover average group BMIs between 18 and 22-

nowhere close to the American regular of 25. For instance, the Okinawa Centenarian Study-which examined a lot more than 1000 centenarians from Okinawa, Japan, over twenty-five years from the mid-1970s to 2001-found that the common BMI of the studied adults was 20.4; The Adventist Health Study-who follow a mainly vegan diet-found an identical result. This twelve-year prospective study of thirty-four thousand middle-aged and elderly Adventists without preexisting illnesses, no background of smoking, cardiovascular system disease, malignancy, or stroke exposed a primary positive relation between a lesser BMI and longevity. An Adventist with a BMI greater than 23 does experience a higher threat of premature death.

Just what exactly can we study from these studies? Based on the data, the utmost acceptable weight generates a BMI of around 22.5, not 25. This implies that the recommended healthful weight for a 5-foot-10-inches adult male is usually between 130 and 160 pounds, and for 5-foot-5-inches adult female is 108 to 135 pounds. That is a large difference from the suitable (not obese) American BMI of 25, which allows 150 pounds for a female and 175 pounds for a guy. Based on the Okinawan and Adventist regular BMI, about 85 per cent of Americans are overweight, not really the 66 per cent based on the NIH. The common American is definitely heavier and sicker than she or he even realizes. All due to the typical

American diet. Hardly anyone can get away its destructive effects. Why else would 90 per cent of everybody older than sixty-five be taking medicines to lessen his or her blood circulation pressure and/or cholesterol? The end result is this: In the event that you eat American meals, you will inevitably develop the illnesses common in America, you shall become overweight, and you will ultimately develop high blood circulation pressure and raised cholesterol (the signs of bloodstream vessel and cardiovascular disease), just like everyone else.

We now contemplate it normal to reduce youthful vigour inside our thirties, carry a supplementary 30 to 40 pounds, live with chronic illness inside our past due forties and fifties, and endure our final years completely reliant on others. But this is simply not normal. This is actually the consequence of a lifelong design of harmful living and misguided info. Instead of dreading deterioration and an increasing number of ailments and medications as we approach later years, we should anticipate enjoying an active existence well into our nineties. This might seem like an outrageous expectation because the majority of us spend eternity eating an unhealthy diet. Today even, too many folks continue to skip the connection between what we consume and how we experience emotionally and actually. Nor can we find out why it appears so difficult to remain at our youthful adult weight.

But it's not as well late.

A high-nutrient diet will certainly reduce your desire to have high-calorie, low-nutrient foods. Within weeks, your taste buds will change, and you'll weary in the processed foods you once believed you could by no means live without. You'll experience more satisfied consuming fewer calorie consumption than you were consuming before. The result is lasting health and long term weight loss. So a lot of my visitors have dropped 100 pounds or even more following my suggestions; they have dropped that much within twelve months, and they have held that weight off for a long time.

THE FINISH of Dieting goes a step beyond Intuitive eating. Not merely does it solution why eating health- completely often appears so difficult, it empowers you with the desire and capability to do so. In the next pages, I talk about the technology and the solutions behind how exactly to rid yourself once and for all of the meals addictions sabotaging your wellbeing. I construct an easy-to-follow eating system you start with a fourteen-day group of easy-to-make, delicious meals that will steadily transform your food preferences, while concurrently recalibrating your palate. I guide your meal options through the first section of the program, so you don't need to think or be concerned in what you're eating-you can merely eat tasty dishes manufactured from fantastic health-assisting foods. In the next area of the programme, I flood the body with nutrition to heal and detoxify it, using very foods in an effort to promote wellness and longevity. By completing and sticking with the program, your BMI shall fall below 22.5 and stay there for the others you will ever have. A diet can just be looked at successful if the meals you eat helps longevity and protect you against cardiovascular disease, stroke, dementia, and malignancy. This nutritarian diet design is the just dietary and nutritional system that guarantees dramatic excess weight reduction without calorie counting. Additionally, it is the just dietary and nutritional plan that explains how to drive back disease while simultaneously significantly increasing your lifespan. Your threat of a coronary attack and/or stroke will almost disappear, and your threat of tumour can plummet by a lot more than 90 per cent, while your daily life expectancy can boost by two decades. Incredible statements, yes, but that is a reality with substantial scientific support. I've observed such outcomes for a lot more than twenty-five years. Forget calorie consumption. The trick of living well is about micronutrients. Eating healthfully and consuming the proper assortment and quantity of nutrients outcomes in consistent, long-term health benefits. Getting healthful and maintaining well balanced, healthful weights are achieved just by concentrating on the dietary quality of your meal. Contrary to standard thinking, it isn't just how much you take in that determines your body weight; it's everything you eat.

Nutritional quality determines your mental, physical, and psychological health-from brain function and an elevated disease fighting capability to happiness and physical well-being. The primary criterion you should think about when choosing what things to eat is which foods are most favourable to your long-term survival. A diet plan style incorporating longevity- advertising foods enables you to try out all sorts of delicious quality recipes, which allows you to continue this new method of eating through the entire rest you will ever have. Any diet you adopt temporarily only results in short-term benefits because eventually your body and your weight change back to the diet you will remain in the long term. I want to repeat that again: Whatever you adopt temporarily just begets temporary outcomes, and fluctuating your body weight up and down isn't life- span favourable. People often view diet programs as a belief program, picking the one which is most closely aligned with their dietary philosophy or food preferences. They often criticize any system that conflicts with these choices. Real science, however, does not have any philosophy or predetermined agenda; it simply flows inexorably from the preponderance of the data. Are you a scientific thinker? Do you want to view reality and allow chips to fall with the data? Remember: Food choices are learned and may be changed.

We have cared for a lot more than 10 thousand people, the majority of whom set foot in my own office unhappy, sick, and overweight. That they had tried each and every dietary craze without achievement. After following my plan, they found out the superior health they always wanted and dropped the weight they always dreamed of losing. Even better, it was kept by them off. For the very first time in their lives, that they had a feeding on the style that didn't keep them starving or unsatisfied. Most of all, they were in a position to stop acquiring their medicines, which had become unneeded.

In the last three decades, I've reviewed a lot more than twenty thousand scientific tests on human nutrition. For this reason, I can state with certainty that is usually the place and today is the period to begin your wellbeing revival. I've seen the results of this plan doing his thing on a large number of people with a wide variety of diseases and health issues, from migraines and allergies to cardiovascular disease and diabetes. The end result is, it functions. Nutritional excellence may be the most effective way to discover long term healthy weight reduction, prevent and invert disease, and end a few of today's most chronic degenerative illnesses.

Your body is a self-therapeutic machine when you supply it with an optimal nutritional environment, and the information presented in this book is the quickest and most effective way to create that environment. In case you have high blood circulation pressure, high cholesterol, diabetes, cardiovascular disease, indigestion, headaches, asthma, exhaustion, body aches, or discomfort- or if you would like to avoid yourself from developing these chronic conditions-this may be the arrange for you. This fresh diet style can allow you in order to avoid angioplasty, bypass medical procedures, and other invasive methods. In the event that you aren't however ill, it could make sure you do not have heart episodes, strokes, or dementia in your old age. It can reduce and eventually get rid of your need for prescription drugs. In short, it can allow you to optimize your health and potentially save your life. And it could do all this while raising the enjoyment you get from meals.

A lot of you have this publication because you would like to lose weight. I wish to assure you that you'll lose all of the weight that you would like, even if diet programs have failed you previously. This is usually the most reliable weight-loss plan ever, and the email address details are permanent, not temporary. Equally essential may be the protection from severe diseases in your own future that this plan gives. The most efficient healthcare is self-care. Medicines and doctors can't grant you superb health insurance and protect you from disease and suffering. Almost every doctor does know this. The dietary excellence I explain in the following can prevent and actually reverse most medical complications within three to half a year. That is a bold state, but the facts- supported by scientific research-display that lots of the tragedies we encounter in today's world are the consequence of nutritional folly. While weight reduction is important, it isn't our main objective. It is an enjoyable and regular by-product on the path to the principal goal: great health. First-class health is definitely marked by an exceedingly long and fairly disease-free lifespan, and countless research reveals that individuals with superior wellness are thin. By teaching you how exactly to achieve superior health, your ideal weight will normally follow. You will understand the physical cravings that trigger overeating, along with the psychological factors that will help you switch this pattern of usage. Applying the info in this reserve to your life can help you create new, healthy behaviours that may eventually become effortless. You will finally maintain control of your health destiny.

This plan will not include counting calories, measuring food portion sizes, or weighing. It doesn't depend on gimmicks or fads. You can end searching for that magic answer since there is no magic remedy. No reddish berry ketones. No green coffees. No purple tulip nectar or dark salt from the white cliffs of Dover. Actually, we almost always, later on, discover that the merchandise that gave us wish was simply hype and that searching for a magic pill causes harm. Whenever a supplement or medicine doesn't meet up with your nutritive requirements, it really is typically toxic and may enhance the damage the effect of a toxic diet.

As we struggled with these issues, we started to explore a few of the popular literature that suggested a 180-level departure from dieting. It proposed a means of consuming that allowed for just about any and all meals choices, regardless of nutrition. Our preliminary reactions were extremely sceptical, if not down- correct rejecting. We reacted with self-righteous indignation. How could we, as nutritionists (authorized dietitians), trained to consider the connections between nourishment and health, sanction a means of eating that appeared to reject the foundation of our understanding and philosophy?

The struggle continued. Healthy eating plans did not help people maintain long-term weight control; the "nutritional waste strategy" was a dangerous choice. The suggestion to ignore nutrition and disregard the way the body seems in response to eating "whatever you want" discount rates the respect for one's body that comes combined with the gift of life. Finally, we resolved the conflict by developing the process of intuitive consumption. This book may be a bridge between its growing movement against diet and the medical community. While the anti-diet movement avoids dieting and blames body acceptance (thankfully), it often doesn't address health risks. How can you reconcile the problems of forbidden foods but still eat healthy, without dieting? We will let you know how in this post.

In case you are like most of our customers, you are tired of dieting but at the same time terrified of eating. Most of our customers feel uncomfortable within their bodies, but don't understand how to change. Intuitive eating provides a new way of eating that is ultimately hassling free and healthy for the brain and body. It really is an activity that frees the chains of the diet (which can only cause deprivation, rebellion and weight gain in extension). This means getting back again to your roots-trusting the body and its signals.

Intuitive eating cannot only change the relationship with food; it can change your daily life.

Intuitive Feeding on includes the principles of mindful eating; in addition, it has a broader philosophy, addressing the problems of cognitive distortions and psychological eating. It includes seeing realization as a central point in consumption, physical activity/movement in relation to feeling good, rejecting the mentality of the diet, using nutritional information without judging and respecting the body, regardless of how you feel about your shape. Intuitive nutrition is undoubtedly a dynamic procedure that integrates the tuning of the brain, body and meals. For those with feeding problems, conscious and intuitive feeding can help facilitate normal feeding.

CHAPTER 1:

HITTING THE DIET BOTTOM

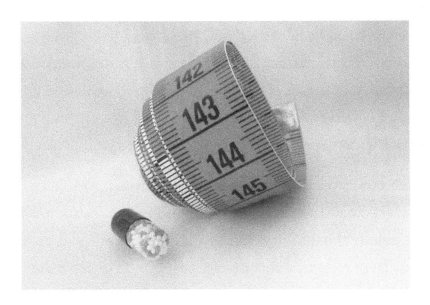

I just can't get on with another diet plan; you are my last resort." Sandra has been on a diet her entire existence and has understood that she could no longer support a single diet program. She had been with all of them, Atkins, Dukan, The Area, South Beach, grapefruit diet ... too many diets for the details. Sandra was a professional on a diet. Initially, the diet was fun, even stimulating. "Usually, I thought this diet will be different right now."

So the routine would be reloaded with every fresh diet, every summer. But the lost weight would eventually be recovered as an undesirable tax bill.

Sandra had hit bottom in the diet plan. At this point, however, I was even more obsessed with meals and her body than ever. She felt silly. "I would have managed and controlled this in the past." What he did not understand was that the dietary procedure had been carried out. Dieting made her even more worried about meals. Diet had made enemy meals. The acquired diet made his experience guilty when he did not consume dietary foods (although she was not officially on a diet). Dieting experienced slowed her metabolism.

Sandra took years to understand that the diet does not work (yes, she knew the emerging idea that the diet does not work, but usually thought it would be different). Some experts and consumers recognize the premise that fast diets don't work: it is difficult for a country of people who are enthusiastic about their bodies to think that even a "practical diet" is often useless. Sandra has been hooked by the interpersonal mythology of the modern age group, the "great hope of diet", for most of her lifestyle since her first diet program at the age of fourteen. At thirty, Sandra felt trapped: she still wanted to lose weight and was uncomfortable in her body. While Sandra couldn't bear the very thought of another diet plan, she didn't understand that the majority of her food problems were actually due to her dieting. Sandra was also discouraged and angry-"I understand everything about diets." Certainly, she could recite calorie consumption and fat grams, just like a walking dietary data source. This is the big warning of losing excess weight and avoiding it usually isn't a problem of understanding. If all we had to have a normal weight was to understand food and nutrition, most people in the United States would not be overweight. The information is easily available. (Take any women's magazine, and you will find abundant diet plans and comparisons with meals).

In addition, the more you try to follow the diet, the more you will fall (it certainly hurts to never succeed in case you have done the best). The best description due to this effect is distributed by John Foreyt, Ph.D., one of the leading professionals of diet psychology. He compared it to a Chinese puzzle (the hollow straw cylindrical puzzle, in which an index finger is placed on each end). The more you try to get out, the more pressure you will exert, the harder it will be to escape the puzzle. Instead, you find yourself locked up in a narrower place ... caught ... frustrated.

SYMPTOMS OF DIET PLAN BACKLASH

Diet backlash may be the cumulative side-effect of dieting-it could be short-term or chronic, depending on how long one has been dieting. It can only be one or more side effects. When

Sandra got to any office, she already had the traditional symptoms of a violent reaction to the diet. Not only was she tired of following a diet, but she ate less food, but she also had problems losing weight during her new diet attempts. Additional symptoms include:

a. The simple contemplation of starting a diet causes desires and cravings for "sinful" and "fatty" foods, such as ice cream, chocolate, biscuits, etc.

b. When you quit a diet, go overeating and feel guilty. One research indicated that post- dieting binges happen in 49 per cent of most individuals who end a diet.

c. Have low self-esteem with meals. It's understandable that every diet program taught you never to trust the body or the food you dedicate. Although it may be the procedure for the diet that fails, failure continues to undermine its romantic relationship with food.

d. Since you don't deserve to consume because you're overweight.

e. Reduced duration of the diet. Living on a diet is getting shorter. (It could be indisputable that the Ultra Slim-Fast sales page is "Give us weekly ... and we ..."

f. Last dinner. All diet plans are preceded by foods that you presume not to eat anymore. Food consumption often increases during this period. It can happen with a meal or in a few days. The last supper seems to be the last step before the "nutritional cleansing", almost a farewell party. For a single customer, Marilyn, each meal seemed to be the last. I ate every meal until it filled up uncomfortable since I was terrified that I would never eat again. Once for all reasons! He was on a diet because the first grade exceeded two-thirds of his existence! He experienced provisional fasting intervals and a series of low-calorie diets. As for his body, the diets were just around the corner, so it's best to eat when you can. Any food for Marilyn was a relief from hunger.

g. Social abstinence. Since it is difficult to go on a diet and visit a party or go out for dinner, it is easier to refuse social invitations. At first, social avoidance of food may seem wiser for dieting reasons, but it becomes a big deal. There is often the concern of being able to maintain static control. It is not unusual for this meeting to be strengthened by "maintaining calorie intake or excess grams of fat for the party", which often means eating almost nothing. But by enough time the dieter finds the party, ravenous food cravings dominates and consuming feels very uncontrollable.

h. Sluggish metabolism. Each diet plan shows your body to adjust better to another purposeful starvation (another eating routine arrangement). The digestion backs off as the body utilizes each calorie successfully, as though it were the last. The more extreme the eating routine, the more it will push your body into the endurance condition that diminishes calories. Bolstering your digestion is like filling a fire. Expel the strong wood, and the fire diminishes. Essentially, to build the pace of digestion, we should eat a satisfactory measure of calories; generally, our life structures will redress and back off.

i. Use caffeine to endure the day. Espresso and diet drinks will, in general, be manhandled as a supervisory group to feel fiery while eating pretty much nothing.

j. Eating disorder. At long last, for a few, the rehashed diet is generally the foundation of a dietary problem (going from anorexia nervosa or bulimia to impulsive indulging).

Despite the fact that Sandra felt she could never again follow dieting, she was as yet engaged with the most recent wonder of the Supper. (We frequently meet him each time we see somebody just because.) Truth be told, she ate higher nourishment levels than expected and ate huge numbers of her preferred nourishments (he figured he could never observe these kinds of nourishment again). It seems as though you are arranging a long outing and planning additional garments. The straightforward thought of concentrating on her eating issues put her in the attitude of the pre-diet plan, something normal.

While Sandra essentially started to comprehend the worthlessness of the dieting, she should be slim had not changed, obviously a predicament. She clung to the appeal of honourable American want.

THE PARADOX OF DIETING

Inside our general public, the quest for slenderness (both for wellbeing and physical make-up) has wound up being the call to war of clearly all Americans. Eating an individual nibble of any nourishment that is high in fat or non-healthfully redeemable is generally deserving of a "blameworthy" expression by affiliation. You may be paroled, in any case, for "extraordinary conduct." Good conduct, inside our way of life, implies beginning a crisp eating routine or having incredible aims to abstain from food. Along these lines starts the hardship routine of dieting- the battle of the "bulge and indulge". Rice cakes for seven days, Häagen-Dazs the following.

"I feel remorseful essentially for enabling the staple worker to perceive what I purchase," said another client, who by chance had his trolley loaded with a natural product, vegetables, entire grains, pasta and a little 16 ounces of genuine dessert. It seems as though we were in a state of utilization of the Food Law coordinated by the nourishment mafia. Furthermore, there consistently is by all accounts dieting you can't refuse. Embellishment? No. We are sensible for this discernment.

A report distributed in 1993 in Eating Disorders-The Journal of Treatment and Avoidance found that somewhere in the range of 1973 and 1991, notices for dietary guides (diet nourishments, nourishment decrease helps, and diet programs) expanded practically direct. The analysts likewise referenced that there is absolutely a parallel model at the beginning of utilization issue. It is speculated that the weight of the push on the dietary arrangement (through publicizing spots) for the most part importantly affects the pattern of buyer unsettling influence.

The dieting pressure plan is powered past TV ads. Magazine articles and film content add to the weight of being thin. Fragile cigarette announcements additionally go for the heaviness of the Achilles female heel with titles like Ultra Thin 100, Virginia Slims, and so forth. A Kent cigarette, "Thin Lights", explicitly portrays this push on ladies' physical issues. Your promotion is like that of an industrialist for a decrease in normal weight contrasted with a cigarette, featuring lean depictions: "long", "slight", "light". Obviously, the examples in cigarette ads are especially unpretentious. Obviously, the inside for disease control (CDC) traits and expansion in ladies' smoking to their need to be more slender. Tragically, we have heard ladies ponder in our workplaces who have likewise viewed as smoking again as a guide to getting more fit.

Be that as it may, weight reduction isn't only a worry of ladies (albeit clearly there is extra weight on ladies). The multiplication of business contributions of light lager has planted the seed of body mindfulness in men's considerations; in addition, a fit stomach is desirable over one of brew. It is no occurrence that we have seen the dispatch of magazines focused on men, for example, Males Fitness and Female's Health.

While the quest for slenderness has crossed the sexual orientation boundary, we have sadly brought forth the original of weight onlookers — an upsetting pattern towards new dieting influences the wellness of American youngsters. Stunning exploration has shown that school-age kids are fixating on their weight-an impression of a nation eager about dieting and overabundance weight. The nation over, six-year-olds are getting thinner, scared of putting on weight, and being continuously treated for utilization issue that compromises their wellbeing and development protection. Social strain to shed pounds has bombed in kids.

Not exclusively can eating less junk food work; it is generally the principle issue. Albeit many may follow dieting as a push to lose abundance weight or for wellbeing reasons, the conundrum is clearly that it could cause more damage. This is the thing that our nation must show to the eating routine:

a. Obesity is greater than any time in recent memory in grown-ups and youngsters.

b. Dietary problems are on the ascent.

c. Child weight issues have multiplied in the previous ten years.

d. Despite the way that there are still more without fat and dietary nourishments than previously, just about 66% of grown-ups are hefty or fat.

e. More than one thousand 200 and a lot of fat has just been liposuction from 1982 to 1992. (And as of late accessible review indicated that once a year after a liposuction procedure, fat returned, yet in another area of the body).

f. Diet builds the possibility to increase significantly a greater number of pounds than you have lost!

DIETING INTAKE CANNOT BATTLE BIOLOGY

Diet is a kind of transient yearning. Accordingly, when you are given a principal chance to eat truly, you experience so firmly that you feel wild, an edgy demonstration. With respect to natural yearning, all expectations to design the eating routine and the need to get in shape are temporary and incomprehensibly superfluous. In those concise minutes, we become simply like the voracious man-expending plant in the film Little Store of Horrors, testing to eat-"Feed me, feed me."

While outrageous eating may appear to be crazy and unnatural, it is really a standard reaction to yearning and diet. Notwithstanding, it can frequently be viewed as that eating after the dieting doesn't have "determination" or imperfection in character. Be that as it may, in translating the post-dietary nourishment plan accordingly, it gradually disintegrates fearlessness with nourishment, diet after eating routine. Each infringement of the eating routine arrangement, each nourishment situation that appears to be wild establishes the frameworks for the "diet plan mindset", step by step and diet by diet. The evidently daring arrangement invest more energy following time-transforms into as dumbfounding as the Chinese finger confound. You can't fight science. At the point when your body starves, it should be bolstered. In any case, frequently a weight watcher gripes: "Just on the off chance that I experience determination." Clearly, this isn't just a self-control issue. (In spite of the fact that the splendid tribute from fat misfortune treatment focuses support this lost blame in determination.) When you are not encouraged, you will get fixated on nourishment, regardless of whether on a purposeful eating routine or craving.

You can't count calories, yet eat cautiously for the sake of wellbeing. This is by all accounts the politically right term for "diet" during the 90s. Be that as it may, in any event, for some, it's a similar issue with dinners, with similar side effects.

Keeping away from overabundance fats or sugars, whatever occurs, and subsisting on basically sans fat or starch-free nourishments is basically an eating routine and frequently brings about a lacking eating routine. There are numerous kinds of diets and different sorts of diets. We will investigate your dietary character and meet the Intuitive Eater in the following part.

DIET INCREASES YOUR RISK OF GETTING MORE WEIGHT!

On the off chance that dietary applications were to withstand a similar control as medications, open utilization probably won't be permitted. Envision, for instance, taking asthma to medicate, which improves relaxing for half a month; however, over the long haul; it exacerbates the lungs and relaxing. Will I truly follow an eating routine (a great supposed "reasonable eating routine"), in the event that I realized I could make you put on weight?

Here is a couple of calming research demonstrating that eating less junk food advances weight gain:

a. A gathering of UCLA specialists inspected thirty-one long haul investigated on eating less junk food and figured slimming down is a consistent indicator of overabundance weight gain-up to 66% of the individuals recovered more abundance weight than they dropped (Mann et al., 2007).

b. Research on almost seventeen thousand kids between the ages of nine and fourteen finished up: "... in the long haul, the weight-controlling eating routine isn't just ineffectual, yet could advance weight gain" (Field et al. 2003).

c. People on a high school diet had twice the same number of odds of being overweight than adolescents on dieting regarding a multiyear review. Specifically, toward the start of the examination, individuals on an eating routine don't gauge significantly more than their companions who don't follow dieting. This is a significant detail, provided that individuals on dieting weigh much more, it could be a component of perplexity (which would suggest extra factors, as opposed to counting calories, for example, genetics).

Epic research on more than 2,000 units of twins from Finland, matured 16 to 25 years matured indicated that consuming fewer calories itself, free of hereditary qualities, is impressively connected with quickened fat addition and expanded danger of getting stout (Pietilaineet et al. 2011). Dietary twins, who experienced a solitary purposeful health improvement plan, were just about a few times bound to be overweight than their non-dietary twin partner.

Likewise, the plausibility of unreasonable overweight improved in a portion subordinate way with every dietary occasion.

Studies aside: what did your dietary experiences show you? Numerous people and individuals in the lab state their first dieting plan was straightforward: the pounds basically liquefied away. Yet, that first dietary experience could be the temptation trap, which starts the vain quest for weight decrease through eating routine. We state pointless on the grounds that our bodies are amazingly wise and designed for endurance.

Organically, your body experiences the dieting process predominantly in light of the fact that it is a sort of starvation. Your cells don't comprehend you are intentionally limiting your dinner admission. The body shifts into base endurance mode-digestion diminish, and nourishment needing heighten. What's more, with each diet plan, your body learns and adjusts, which prompts weight gain in expansion. Therefore, many people feel simply like they absolutely are a disappointment; however, it truly is eating less junk food which has bombed them.

CHAPTER 2:

WHAT TYPE OF EATER ARE YOU?

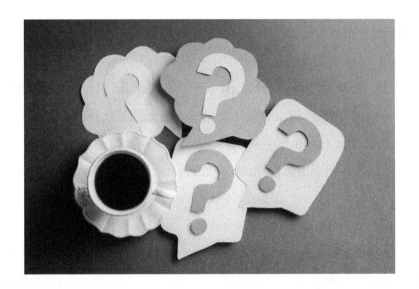

You can continue on a diet and not know! There are many types of eating styles that are actually unconscious types of dieting. Quite a few people have said these were not really on a diet plan- but upon nearer inspection of what and how they consume, they were dieting still!

A good example here's. Ted arrived because he wished to lose excess weight. He said that in his fifty years of life, he had previously only been on four serious diet programs. In examining the titles of publications at work (compulsory overeating texts, consumption of books on ailments, etc.), he said: "You use many serious complications in the diet ... well, I'm not just one of those. Obviously, Ted did not consider himself a dietician, who ate simply with care, but showed that it was an unconscious diet.

Although Ted had not followed an active diet, he was eating at a level where he had almost passed out in the afternoon. The reason: he had been unhappy with his weight! In the morning I chose an intense bicycle trip down a hill, for only an hour. I would go back and have breakfast for a bit. Lunch was usually a salad with iced tea (although it seems healthy, it is too low in carbohydrates). At dinner time, your body will scream for meals. Ted not only had a severe calorie deficit, but he also lacked carbohydrates. Nights become a food party! Ted had the idea that it was previously a "food volume" problem with a solid sweet tooth. The truth is that previously he had an unconscious mentality in the diet that biologically triggered his night diet and his pleasant tooth.

Even Alicia hadn't been on a conscious diet. She never came to lose pounds, but because she wanted to increase her vitality. During the initial program, it became clear that he had problems with food. So they asked him if he had done many diets. She seemed amazed. "How did you know I did billions of diets?" While Alicia claimed to be comfortable with her current fat, she was still at war with food; she did not trust herself with meals. It turns out that Alicia has been on a diet since she was a child. Although he hadn't officially followed a diet, he maintained (and expanded) a couple of dietary guidelines with each diet plan that almost paralyzed her ability to eat normally. We observe this at all times, the hangover from dieting: avoiding certain foods no matter what, feeling uncontrollable as soon as a "sinful" meals are eaten, sense guilty when self-imposed food guidelines are broken (such as for example "Thou shalt not really eat previous to 6 P.M."), and so forth. The unconscious diet usually occurs in the type of meticulous eating habits. There can be an excellent line between feeding on for health insurance and dieting. Notice how actually the frozen diet plan foods such as for example, Lean Cuisine and Excess weight Watchers are placing their focus on health instead of a diet. As long as you participate in some form of the diet, the recipient will eliminate food and body concerns. Whether you are a conscious or unconscious person, the results of the medial side are similar, the diet again, the effect of the eyelashes. It seems like a period in which one eats cautiously, "blowing" it and spending penance with an increase in diet or extremely cautious consumption. In this chapter, we will explore the many diet/nutrition styles to help see what your position is now. Later, you will meet the Intuitive Eater and the intuitive style of food, and the perfect solution is to live without diet programs.

THE EATING PERSONALITIES

To help you clarify your food design style (or diet), we have identified the following key types of eaters that feature distinctive food patterns: the careful eater, the one that makes a professional diet and the eater unconscious. These consuming personalities are exhibited even if they are not officially on a diet. It is possible to have significantly more than one consuming personality, although we find that there is commonly a dominant trait. The chances of your life can also influence or change your personality to eat. For example, a client, a tax attorney, was usually a careful eater, but during the fiscal period of the year, it became the chaotic unconscious eater.

It is possible that it occasionally possesses the intake characteristics described below in the three nuclei that feed on personality. Note this, and if your feed exists in one of these domains most of the time, it's a problem.

Review each character you eat and see which one best reflects your style. By understanding what your position is now, it will be easier to find out how to become an intuitive eater. For example, you may find that you have already been involved in a type of diet and have not even recognized it. Or you can discover features that, without knowing it, work against you.

THE CAREFUL EATER

Cautious consumers are those who tend to be attentive to the food they put into their bodies. Ted was a good example of a careful eater (per day). At the top, accurate eaters look like "ideal" eaters. They are highly aware of nutrition. Externally, they seem oriented towards health and fitness (noble characteristics admired and strengthened in our society).

Style

There is a selection of eating behaviours exhibited by Careful Eater. In an intense moment, Cautious Eater can be distressed for every bite of food allowed in the body. Shopping trips are spent looking at meal labels. Eating out can indicate interrogating the waiter what's in the meals, how maybe the meals prepared-and obtaining assurances that the meals are prepared particularly to the Cautious Eater's liking (not often one speck of essential oil or other excess fat used). What's incorrect with this? Aren't label reading and assertive cafe ordering in the medical interests of some individuals? Of program! However, the difference could be the vigilante force and the ability to forget any defect related to the choice of consumption. Attentive eaters tend to consume less than normal and control the amount of food consumed.

The attentive eater can spend most of his waking hours planning another meal or snack, often worried about eating.

Since Careful Eater is not officially on a diet, your brain punishes all the "harmful", fatty or sugary foods you eat. The Careful Eater can travel the fine line between sincerely thinking about health and eating carefully with respect to body image. Sometimes, Careful Eater is driven by periods or events. For example, some careful eaters are meticulous during weekdays, to make sure they get their "ideal of consumption" to "show off" on the weekends or for the next party. But on weekends they happen 104 times a year: waste can be counterproductive with unwanted weight gain. Consequently, it is not uncommon for a cautious eater to think about starting a diet.

The Problem

There's nothing incorrect with being thinking about the well-being of the body. However, the problem occurs when diligent consumption (almost in contact with the militant) affects a healthy relationship with food and negatively affects the body. Prudent eaters, on closer inspection, resemble a delicate diet style. They can't be on a diet; however, they look into every food scenario.

THE PROFESSIONAL DIETER

People on a professional diet are easier to identify; they are on a perpetual diet. In general, they tried the latest commercial diet, the diet book or the trick to lose weight. Sometimes, the diet is performed in the form of fasting or "reduction".

Professional Dieters understand a whole lot about portions of foods, calories, and "dieting methods," yet the cause they are usually on another diet plan is that the initial one never worked. Today, Professional Dieter can be amply trained in counting carbohydrate grams.

Style

People on a professional diet also have accurate food traits. The difference, however, is that people on a diet chronically, guiding the choice of meals to lose weight, not necessarily for health. When the dieter is not officially on a diet, he generally thinks about the next diet that can be started. He often wakes up wishing this is a good day, the fresh start. While people on a professional diet have a lot of knowledge of diets, they don't serve them well. It is not uncommon to allow them to eat compulsively or participate in the consumption of the Last Supper as soon as a prohibited meal is eaten.

This is because people on a chronic diet really believe that they will no longer eat this food; tomorrow I'm on a diet, tomorrow they start again with a clean slate. Better eat right now; it's the last opportunity. And in addition, the Professional Dieter gets discouraged at the futility of the vicious routine. Diet, lose weight, put on weight, intermittent binges, and back again to dieting.

The Problem

It's very difficult to live in this manner. The Yo-Yo diet helps make losing excess weight more difficult as well as eating healthy. Chronic lack of food usually causes overeating or periodic feeding. For some diet professionals, the frustration of losing weight intensifies so much that they can try laxatives, diuretics and weight loss supplements. And trigger that these "dietary aids" generally don't work, they could try extreme methods like chronic restriction, in the type of anorexia nervosa or bleeding (like nausea after a binge), in the type of bulimia. While anorexia and bulimia are multifactorial and have their roots in psychological problems, a growing body of research suggests that chronic diet is usually a common step towards an eating disorder. One study specifically found that when enough dieters reach the age of fifteen, they are eight times more likely to have problems with an eating disorder than people who don't go on a diet.

THE UNCONSCIOUS EATER

The Unconscious Eater is often engaged in a paired diet, which consists of eating and simultaneously doing another activity, such as watching television and eating, or eating and reading. Due to the subtleties and insufficient awareness, it can become problematic for a person to recognize this eating character. There are numerous subtypes of unconscious eaters.

THE CHAOTIC UNCONSCIOUS EATER

Live a life that is too often programmed, too busy, too many things you can do. The chaotic, consuming design is haphazard; whatever's obtainable will end up being grabbed-vending machine fare, junk food, it'll all perform. Food and diet tend to be vital to this person-just not really in the critical instant of the chaos. Chaotic eaters tend to be so busy putting out fires that have difficulty identifying biological cravings for food until it is fiercely voracious. And in addition, the chaotic eater will go extended periods of time without eating.

THE REFUSE-NOT UNCONSCIOUS EATER

They are vulnerable to the simple existence of food, regardless of whether they are hungry or full. The jars of sweets, the meals at the meetings, the food sitting on the kitchen counter, probably none of them will be overcome. However, most of the time, it is fair; consumers who do not refuse to consume are not aware of what they are consuming or how much they consume. For example, the Reject-Not Eater can actually pick up some candy on the way to the bathroom without being aware of it. Social outings that revolve around meals such as cocktails and festive buffets are particularly difficult for Refuse-Not Eater.

THE WASTE-NOT UNCONSCIOUS EATER

Evaluate meals in dollars. His / her eating travel is frequently influenced by getting just as much as they are able to your money can buy. Waste-Not Eater is particularly inclined to completely clean the plate (and also that of others). It is not unusual for a waste eater not to actually consume the leftovers of children or spouse.

THE UNCONSCIOUS EMOTIONAL EATER

They use food to manage emotions, especially unpleasant feelings such as stress, anger and loneliness. While Emotional Eaters look at their consuming as the problem, it's often a sign of a deeper concern. Consuming behaviours of the Emotional Eater can range between grabbing a bag of chips on stressful occasions to chronic compulsive binges of huge quantities of food.

The problem

Unconscious power, in its many forms, usually be a problem if it translates into persistent excessive consumption (which can simply occur if you are eating instead of being very alert). Remember that somewhere between the first and last bite of meals is where the awareness period actually occurs. Like in "Oh, it's all over!"

For example, have you ever bought a large package of candy in the movies and started consuming it, and then you find that your fingertips suddenly scratch themselves under the empty container?

This is a simple type of unconscious feeding. But unconscious nutrition can also exist at an extreme level, in a relatively altered feeding condition. In this case, the individual is not attentive to what is consumed, why he has started eating, or how he knows about the taste of the food. That is zoning out with meals.

WHEN YOUR EATING PERSONALITY WORKS AGAINST YOU

Finally, the food varieties of Careful Eater, Professional Dieter and Unconscious Eater become an inefficient feeding method, even if at the top they seem to be fine. The perfect solution is for the discouraged consumer: try more with a fresh diet!

At first, the new diet seems stimulating and hopeful, but in the end, the family pounds return. The diet becomes more demanding, and even if you resume your basal consumption personality, you may feel more unpleasant than before. It is because internal dietary guidelines are strengthened with each diet plan. T

hese meal rules often perpetuate the guilt emotions of consumption, even when you are not officially on a diet. Furthermore, the biological ramifications of the diet make it increasingly difficult to have a normal romantic relationship with meals. The Intuitive Eater character, however, can be an exception. It's the only feeding design that doesn't work against you and will help you end chronic diets and yo-yo weight fluctuations.

INTUITIVE EATER INTRODUCTION

Intuitive eaters march with their signs of internal hunger and eat regardless of what they choose without feeling guilty or an ethical dilemma. The intuitive eater can be an independent eater. However, it is increasingly difficult to become an unaltered eater in today's health-conscious society considering the bombardment of communications on food, food and weight by advertisers, the press and medical researchers. When we explained the basic feeding characteristics of Intuitive Eater to its customers, it is surprising how often we will hear the answer: "This is how my partner eats." This or how my boyfriend eats. "When we ask what the person's weight and romantic relationship is with food, the answer is: "No problem!" Consider small children. Intuitive, natural eaters will be practically free of social messages about meals and body image. Toddlers possess innate wisdom of meals, in the event that you don't hinder it. They don't eat predicated on dieting guidelines or health, yet study after research shows that if you allow a toddler consumes spontaneously; he'll eat what he requirements when given free usage of food. (This is most likely the toughest point for a concerned mother or father to do- to release and trust that children have an innate capability to eat!)

This is true even when food for food, food for little tykes is apparently a father's nightmare. Experts found that calorie intake was highly variable in confirmed foods; However, it has been balanced over time. However, many parents assume that their children cannot properly regulate their diet.

As a result, parents often adopt coercive strategies in an attempt to ensure that the child eats a nutritionally sufficient diet. But a previous study by Birch and his colleagues indicates that these control strategies are countered. In addition, Birch notes that "parents' attempts to regulate their children's feeding have been reported more regularly by obese adults than by normal-weight adults." Likewise, Duke University psychologist Philip Costanzo, PhD found that unwanted weight in school-age children was closely related to the level at which parents sought to limit their children's food. Actually, well-meaning parents hinder Intuitive Eating. Whenever a mother or father attempts to overrule a child's organic eating cues, the nagging problem gets worse, not better.

A parent, who feeds a kid every time a hunger signal is heard and who stops feeding when the infant demonstrates he's had enough, may play a robust role in the original development of Intuitive Feeding on. Indeed, the innovative role of the therapist and dietician offered by Ellyn Satter has shown that, in the event that the parents of obese children cool down and allow them to consume without the pressure of their parents, the children will ultimately eat much less. Why? The child begins to listen and understand his internal signs of hunger and satiety. The child also knows that he will use food.

According to Satter, "children deprived of food so that they can lose weight, worry about food, fear they don't have enough to eat and are susceptible to overeating if they get the chance." We have found that this is accurate for dieters too. Limited to adults, the intuitive drinking process has been buried over a long period, often years and years. Instead of relaxing a father's pressure, this decrease in pressure should be the result of inside and against the myth of society about dieting and distorted body worship.

Fortunately, we all have the natural ability to eat intuitively; It has simply been suppressed, especially with the diet. This book specializes in showing you exactly how to wake the intuitive eater in you.

HOW YOUR INTUITIVE EATER GETS BURIED

As toddlers get yourself a little older, the mixed messages start to creep in-from the early influences of the Saturday morning food commercial, to the well-meaning mother or father who coaxes his kid to "Clean your plate." The assault won't stop if you're a kid. There are many external forces that impact our eating, that may include additionally bury Intuitive Eating.

DIETING

You have already seen the damage from a chronic diet, which includes, among others:

a. Increase in excessive consumption
b. Decreased metabolic rate.
c. Greater concern about meals.
d. Increase the emotions of deprivation.
e. A greater sense of failure
f. Reduced feeling of willpower.

This only serves to erode your confidence in food and prompts you to rely on external sources to guide your diet (one diet, one diet and enough time of the day, food rules, etc.). The more you head to external resources to "judge" if your consuming is in balance, the additional removed you feel from Intuitive Eating. Intuitive Eating depends on your inner cues and signals.

EAT HEALTHY MESSAGES OR DIE

Messages about healthy eating are everywhere, from nonprofit healthcare organizations to food companies promoting the medical benefits of their unique item. The inherent message? Everything you consume can improve your wellbeing. Conversely, take one incorrect move (bite), and you're one step nearer to the grave. Is usually this an exaggeration? No. For example, a 1994 press release published by the Harvard College of Public Health mentioned that the consumption of trans-fatty acids (inside margarine) could cause thirty thousand deaths each year in the United States due to cardiovascular disease. That sort of message can easily keep you feeling guilty for consuming the "incorrect" kind of meals and feeling puzzled in what you should eat.

Magazines and newspapers have also significantly increased their protection of food and well-being. A food publisher, Joe Crea, of an important metropolitan newspaper, the Orange County Register (California), said that in a period of six to 12 months (1987-1993) his stories about food multiplied by five. Of nearly eight hundred food stories, two hundred had been linked to health problems. Although there is absolutely no doubt that everything you eat can affect your health, exponential coverage of the press has been offered as a channel for the development of food paranoia in the purchaser, particularly in the diet. Joe Crea agrees: "Open the newspaper, visit a good story about cheesecake and, at the same time, another piece on how eating too much will make you gain weight. Place the incompatible player. Are we saying you should ignore the virtues of healthy intake? Of course not. However, if you have a diet adapted to your diet, the burst of "healthy eating" messages can make you feel more guilty about the foods you choose to eat. Obesity and Wellness reported a study of 2,075 adults in Florida that revealed that 45% of adults felt guilty after eating the foods they liked. (Remember that this study was carried out to reflect common American demographics. These "guilt-by- eating" figures would probably be higher if performed on dieters.) Women could be particularly guilty. A Gallup poll by the American Dietetic Association showed that women feel more guilty than men for the foods they eat (44 per cent versus 28 per cent). Could this be because females diet more often than men? Or because ladies are usually the prospective of health communications and food advertisements (consider the number of women's magazines). Women will be primarily responsible for decisions relating to family health care and will often also be responsible for food and nutritional problems; They serve as the main objective.

We have found that establishing a healthy diet or diet as a short priority in the intuitive feeding process is counterproductive. We initially ignore nutrition, as it interferes with the relearn process of an intuitive eater. Nutrition heresy? No. Food can be respected and honoured. It simply cannot be the first priority when you've been on a diet for a lifetime. Or consider it this way; in case you have focused all your attention on the diet, does it help you? The many nutritious diet programs (absolute) may become embraced as another type of diet.

CHAPTER 3:

INTUITIVE EATING STANDARDS: SUMMARY

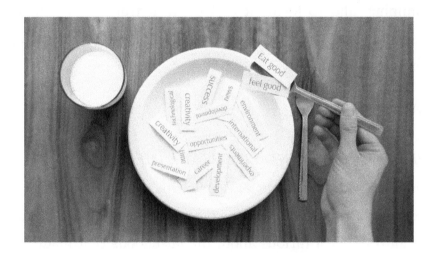

J ust once he vows to dispose of the diet and supplant it with an activity focused on intuitive nourishing, is he considering escaping jail from abundance weight variances and food fixations? In this part, we will present the fundamental ideas of intuitive sustaining: a preview of every idea, with an examination study or two. The most significant aftereffect of every customer referenced was that of acquiring a sound association with dinners and their bodies. By following ten intuitive eating ideas, you will standardize your sentimental association with food. A focus on weight reduction must be set aside for later. On the off chance that your present pounds offer came about because of getting withdrawn together with your inward insight about eating, and subsequently, of tuning back into this intelligence, weight reduction happens, along these lines be it. Assuming, by the by, you are as of now keeping your set point fat through the action of limiting, overeating, confining, and so forth, at that point, it truly is particularly essential that you put weight to decrease on the storage compartment burner.

GUIDELINE ONE:

DECLINES THE MENTALITY OF THE DIETARY PLAN

Dispense with diet books and magazine articles that give you the bogus any desire for getting more fit rapidly, effectively and for all time. Feel furious about the falsehoods that made you sense that you had flopped each time a new diet quit working and you recovered all your weight. On the off chance that you enable a little want to demand that a crisp and better diet might be hiding close by, it will keep you from abstaining from rediscovering the intuitive diet.

For quite a while, we have sought after one diet plan for another, enabling the most stylish trend to direct what, how much, and when to eat. This inflexible way of life of limitation and hardship can bring about a dangerous association with food. The initial step on the intuitive sustenance scale is, for the most part, to depend on your impulses with respect to food decisions.

GUIDELINE TWO:

RESPECT YOUR HUNGER

Keep your body organically encouraged with adequate vitality and sugars. Else you can bring about base travel to indulge. When you reach the top appetite, all aims of moderate, conscious eating are passing and unessential. Seeing how to respect this first organic sign units the phase for revamping trust with yourself and dinners.

While most diets need you to object to a growling stomach, intuitive nutrition renews your body's signals. You'll make sense of how to be increasingly aware of your food yearnings and how precisely to react appropriately to it before you feel hungry. Attempt this in the home: Before each dinner, rate your level of yearning, record a couple of internal signals that you saw, and enough time of day. Do this for week by week, and you'll are more in order together with your hunger, and furthermore which foods convey dependable vitality and the ones that are quickly catching fire and convey short-lived satiety.

GUIDELINE THREE:

MAKE PEACE WITH FOOD

Call a détente; quit the food battle! Give unconditional approval to food. In the event that you illuminate yourself that you can't or shouldn't have a particular food, it can bring about serious feelings of hardship that incorporate with wild longings and, regularly, gorging. At the point when you at last "give up" to your illegal foods, eating will be acquainted with such force, it, for the most part, results in Last Supper overeating and overpowering blame.

Intuitive eating solicits that you forsake the idea from awful and the great food. That system energizes an unsafe 'win big or bust by any stretch of the imagination' attitude that may bring about longings for 'taboo' foods, joined by gorging and a rush of self-hatred and disgrace. Intuitive eating advances the hypothesis that food ought to be viewed as an actual existence upgrading experience.

GUIDELINE FOUR:

CHALLENGE THE MEALS POLICE

Shout a boisterous "basically no" to contemplations in your mind that proclaim you're "extraordinary" for eating under one thousand calories or "horrendous" in light of the fact that you ate a touch of chocolate cake. THE MEALS LAW

AUTHORIZATIONS POLICE, the nonsensical rules that dieting has created. The police headquarters is certainly housed somewhere down in your mind, and its own amplifier yells ominous points, sad expressions, and blame inciting arraignments. Pursuing the suppers Police aside is a significant advance in time for Intuitive Eating. An escalated mental housekeeping and reframing disposition toward suppers are pivotal. Watch any food law authorization considerations you may have, such as "I was poor today" or "I shouldn't eat that." Resist the possibility that your food alternatives characterize it and the value it brings to the world. Pay special mind to people who might be deliberately or unwittingly showing a food police mindset, at that point talk about your intuitive eating way of thinking with them and have them to help you by hushing up about their terrible remarks.

GUIDELINE FIVE:

FEEL YOUR FULLNESS

Tune in for the body flags that let you realize that you are not any hungrier. Pay heed to the signs that show that you're effectively full. Interruption in the focal point of suppers or nibble and have yourself the manner in which the food tastes, and what your present completion level is.

The other side of regarding your appetite is to regard when you're full. Since diet programs limit what, when, and exactly the amount you expend, it's easy to get detached from the internal signs that transmission satiety. At the point when you practice intuitive expending you take up a feast with a lesser degree of food yearnings and in a mentality which enables you to turn out to be increasingly fragile to prompts that you're full. In addition, you comprehend that you could refuel at whatever point you're ravenous once more, and you won't encounter constrained to clean your plate totally. Evaluate this at home: Make utilization of a satiety scale all through suppers to prepare your brain to address signs of satiety. Record perceptions of how you are feeling and all that you ate. This can help decide when to leave the fork and let the dinners actually feel supported and empowered.

GUIDELINE SIX:

REVEAL THE SATISFACTION FACTOR

JAPAN has the knowledge to keep joy as you of their objectives of sound living. Inside our anger to be thin and sound, we regularly ignore likely the essential presents of presence the happiness and fulfilment, which can be inside the eating experience. At the point when you take in what you need, in a domain that is welcoming, the fulfilment you infer is incredible power in helping you are feeling fulfilled and content. By giving this experience to yourself, you will see that it takes essentially less food to pick; you've had "enough."

Intuitive eating urges you to perceive foods that really cause you to feel great all through supper, yet a short time later, as well. You will find yourself floating towards and time for the foods that produce you feel your absolute best. Besides to relishing suppers and eating groceries that taste extraordinary and make you feel incredible, you can connect the entirety of your faculties: slow down, acknowledge what kind of food looks, regard how it achieved your plate, inhale every one of the fragrances, and eat inside a domain that appears to be acceptable expedite the plants and candles-and with people who light you up.

GUIDELINE SEVEN:

ADAPT TOGETHER TO YOUR EMOTIONS WITHOUT NEEDING FOOD

Discover approaches to solace and simplicity, sustain, occupy, and illuminate your passionate worries without utilizing food. Stress, depression, weariness, and outrage are sentiments a large portion of us experience all through presence. Everyone has its trigger, and every offer its own conciliation. Suppers won't fix these sentiments. It could comfort for the present moment, divert from the distress, or really numb you directly into a food aftereffect. However, food won't solve the problem. In the event that anything, eating for an enthusiastic yearning is just going to make you feel more awful after some time.

You'll, in the end, need to adapt to the wellspring of the feeling, alongside the distress of overeating. Indeed, food could be encouraging, yet that delight just keeps going insofar as the food. A short time later, anything that was eating you stays, covered under food, perhaps now offered with a piece of blame and disgrace. Intuitive eating urges you to perceive whether you're sense on edge, exhausted, desolate, tragic, or irate and look for a veritable arrangement. Get a walk, call a dear companion, practice reflection or yoga, get a remedial back rub, read a composed book, or make in a diary. You'll comprehend you're reacting appropriately when the reaction empowers you to feel good, not more terrible.

GUIDELINE EIGHT:

RESPECT YOUR BODY

Acknowledge your hereditary outline. Just for the most part in light of the fact that an individual with a footwear size of eight wouldn't ordinarily foresee reasonably to crush directly into a size six, it truly is correspondingly useless (and horrendous) to have a comparable desire regarding the matter of body size. Regard the body, so you can encounter better about who you are. It's difficult to dismiss the dietary plan attitude in the event that you are ridiculous and excessively pivotal of the body shape. Our varieties are our superpowers, but we live in a world that idealizes a cut body type. The possibility that individuals can profoundly change our life structures is typically unreasonable and ridiculous. Intuitive eating troubles you to grasp your hereditary plan set handy expectations, and praise your uniqueness. Evaluate this in the home: Anytime you catch yourself contrasting the body with someone else's, react as you'll if a buddy said something practically identical regarding themselves.

GUIDELINE NINE:

EXERCISE-FEEL THE DIFFERENCE

Disregard activist exercise. Just get dynamic and experience the distinction. Move your concentrate to how it appears to go your body, as opposed to the fat consuming limit impact of the activity. On the off chance that you focus on how you are feeling from working out, such as empowered, it could have the effect between turning up for an energetic morning hour's walk and striking the rest caution. If when you stirred, your solitary target is to lose abundance weight, rarely do you get an inspiring component at that time of period. People who practice intuitive benefiting from appreciating practice since it gives them vitality improves their inclination, advances self-adequacy, and makes them experience solid, adaptable, and dexterous. Preparing isn't about which movement will consume off the most calories, however rather about which action might be the best time and stimulating. It's another exemplary instance of the manner in which the fulfilment factor could make propensities stick. The exercise you appreciate is an exercise that you're bound to do it once more, creating the force that drives feasible, long haul bliss.

GUIDELINE TEN:

RESPECT YOUR HEALTHY AND SOFT FOOD

Choose foods that respect your prosperity and taste buds while making you feel better. Comprehend that you don't have to eat a perfect diet to be invigorating. You won't all of a sudden get yourself a supplement lack, or put on weight in one bite, one food, or one day of eating. It's what you normally eat after some time that issues. Progress, not so much flawlessness, is what makes a difference. Recognizing how your prosperity impacts the wealth, you will ever have shallow known purposes behind health objectives and grounds your thought processes in what is important: your individual qualities. Getting the point of view on why health is significant can assist you with the understanding that no supper or chomp could represent the moment of truth your self-esteem. Adjust your prosperity to your aspirations, and you will be significantly progressively inspired to develop rehearses that help your day by day life objectives.

AN ACTIVITY WITH GREAT REWARDS

Numerous people have been disappointed with their association with food and their bodies. Many experienced endeavoured either formal or casual dieting and had encountered disappointment and gloom. By learning the ideas of Intuitive Consuming and putting them to work, many will find an extending of the evaluation of life and quality about eating. You can go as well!

CHAPTER 4:

AROUSING THE INTUITIVE EATER: STAGES

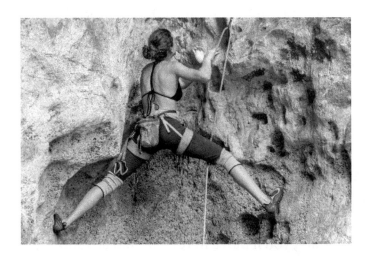

The journey to Intuitive Eating is like going for a cross-district climbing trip. Before you really tie without anyone else climbing boots, you'd have to recognize what's in store all through your outing. While a road map is viable, it doesn't disclose what you'll be enough prepared, such as trail conditions, atmosphere, special touring detects, the kind of garments to put on, etc. The goal of this part is, for the most part, to help you comprehend what to envision all through your outing to Intuitive Eating.

Regardless of whether it's strolling or relearning an unmistakably all the more fulfilling eating plan, you will continue through numerous phases in transit. The amount of time that you should remain static in a specific stage is certainly a factor and amazingly individualized. For example, crossing new climbing trails relies on how physically fit you are, the way you adapt to worry with a new path, exactly how much time you have to climb, and the choice of climbing trails. In like manner, your adventure back again to Intuitive Eating relies on how protracted you've been dieting, how emphatically settled in your everyday diet believing is the means by which long you've been utilizing suppers to deal with life, that you are so arranged to confide in yourself, and that you are so prepared to put weight decrease on the storage compartment burner and see how to turn into an Intuitive Eater the essential objective.

Now and again, you'll move in reverse and advances among the stages. In the event that you recognize that is an ordinary segment of the procedure, it can assist you with continuing without inclination that you will fall away from the faith or not so much gaining ground. Think about this circumstance: You are on a mobile path and experience a fork in the road that is difficult to unravel together with your path map. Do you go legitimately to one side or left? You consider for quite a while and pick to go remaining. While strolling, you place something you've in no way, shape or form seen previously, a sparkling green caterpillar shimmying up a purple bloom. A couple of activities ahead, you find a novel fowl. In any case, a couple of strategies past these wonders of character are a huge rock flagging that you locate an inappropriate course. You pivot, return to the fork, and think about the other course. Was this temporary re-routing an exercise in futility?

No! So also, in connection to Intuitive Eating, you will require numerous turns and test out new contemplations and practices. You may locate that subsequent to creating recognizable advancement, and you return to old procedures are terrible and unfulfilling. In any case, such as gaining "an inappropriate" course on the grand trekking trail, you'll see that outings into matured expending examples can be used as learning encounters. (Numerous climbers wouldn't ordinarily scold themselves to be uncertain of what direction to take; rather, they'd be grateful for the disclosures of character that a blocked course offered.) It's imperative that you help yourself out and welcome the preparation that turns out from experience. This procedure includes originating from a position of interest rather than a position of judgment, along these lines whatever you do; don't crush yourself up intellectually!

Intuitive Eating is very not equivalent to dieting. Dieters, for the most part, get disappointed on the off chance that they don't follow the dietary plan way decisively as endorsed. We've seen numerous a relentless dieters simply have an off-base change at one feast, be critical for that error, and "blow" the dietary plan for that day time or end of the week or in reality longer! Recall that the outing to Intuitive Eating is typically a procedure, loaded up with good and bad times, un-like dieting where in actuality the regular desire is unquestionably direct advancement (losing a specific measure of abundance weight in a specific time span).

The road to Intuitive Eating is like obtaining a long haul common store. Over the long haul, you will see an arrival on speculation, paying little mind to the everyday vacillations of the money markets. It is customary and anticipated. How amusing that individuals have been prepared that, in financial matters, the everyday changes in the cash markets are typical, and once in a while is there a moment get-rich fix, yet, in the multibillion-dollar, a year pounds misfortune business, "get slender quick" might be the main target for accomplishment. We are contributed, rather, in helping you give harmony to your expending presence and self-perception. In connection to this objective, remember Webster's portrayal of procedure: "a continuous advancement including numerous alterations" and "a particular way to deal with accomplishing something, including various advances or activities by and large."

Much like any procedure, it's essential that you remain centred in, and develop from the numerous experiences you will experience. Assuming, in any case, you focus on the result (which for some, people is fat or the number of pounds lost), it could make you experience overpowered and debilitated, and wrap up disrupting the strategy. Rather, if your air conditioning information little changes in transit and worth the preparation encounters (that may in some cases be disappointing), it can assist you with adhering to the Intuitive Eating course and push ahead. When you truly become an Intuitive Eater, you will consistently check out your inward insight, and you may feel better on a basic level, body, and soul.

Now, we feel it is important to explain the issue of the mission for weight reduction. For a few, the body will return to its normal abundance weight level, which might be not exactly your present pounds and remain there. To watch if this relates to you, ask yourself the following inquiries: Perhaps you have routinely destroyed from agreeable totality level? Perform you routinely gorge when you're getting arranged for the following diet (understanding that there will turn into a ton of foods you won't be allowed to eat on the dietary plan)? Perform your gorge as an adapting framework in troublesome events or to fill period when you're exhausted? Maybe you have been impervious to work out?

Do you only exercise in the event that you are dieting? Do you skip foods or hold back to eat until you're insatiably hungry, possibly to find that you indulge when you at long last expend?

Do you are feeling remorseful; either when you indulge or when you take in all that you call a "poor food," which results in all the more overeating? If you addressed "yes" for a few of the vast majority of these inquiries, after that all things considered, your present weight might be more prominent than the weight the body is intended to keep up. Furthermore, it is likely you will have the option to return to your common, sound weight, because of this procedure. Be that as it may, recall, weight decrease should be put on the storage compartment burner. In the event that you focus on weight reduction, it'll meddle with your ability to settle on decisions predicated on your intuitive signs.

When you've surrendered the pointlessness of dieting perpetually, you'll wind up eating far fewer suppers with a craving to see customary movement in your day by day life. You'll find that the body feels so far superior when your midsection isn't stuffed, at whatever point your muscle tissue is conditioned, just as your heart is coordinate. You will likewise find that as your contemplations about your eating and body begin to transform, you will encounter an all the more loosening up feeling, rather than the incessant foundation stress that weaving machines each supper decision. Nonetheless, if you keep on focusing on weight decrease as the objective, you'll get tangled up in the matured diet-attitude figuring, which won't serve you.

Throughout the years, we've seen our people continue through a five-organize movement in figuring out how to be an Intuitive Eater. The following segment can assist you with getting an idea of what things to expect inside your very own adventure.

STAGE ONE: READINESS-HITTING DIET PLAN BOTTOM

This is the place numerous individuals start. You are agonizingly conscious that each attempt to get in shape is made in "falling flat." You are wary of esteeming every day predicated on whether the level is as a rule up or down a pound or two (or on the off chance that you indulged your prior day). You envision and stress over dinners constantly. You talk the prohibitive food visit "Just in the event that I didn't have to watch my overabundance weight, I could expend that," or "I encountered two treats I truly was awful today."

As of now, your weight might be higher than any time in recent memory, or, without significantly over-weight, you lose and increase five or ten pounds to such an extent and rapidly as you wash your garments in addition to they get filthy again! You have lost contact with organic food longings and satiety signals. You have overlooked all that you truly prefer to expend and rather eat all that you figure you "should" eat. Your association with dinners has built up a poor tone, and you fear to eat the foods you like since you're apprehensive it'll be difficult to stop.

At the point when you yield to the enticement of illegal foods, it's normal to indulge them, since you are feeling remorseful. However, you earnestly pledge you won't ever eat them again.

It's not bizarre to get that you take into comfort, occupy, or even numb yourself from your very own emotions. On the off chance that that is the situation, you will feel that an incredible evaluation offers been blurred by obsession thinking about suppers and by careless expending.

The self-perception is negative-you don't simply like the manner in which you show up and feel inside your body, and confidence is reduced. You have found from your experience that dieting won't work-you have arrived in a desperate predicament and experience stuck, debilitated, and disheartened.

This stage proceeds until you select that you will be troubled eating and living along these lines you will be prepared to accomplish something positive about it.

Your first contemplations may veer toward finding another diet to determine your issues. Yet, very quickly, you comprehend that you can't do that one until kingdom come. On the off chance that that is the place you find yourself, you at that point are set up for the method that will empower you to get back again to eating intuitively.

STAGE TWO: EXPLORATION-CONSCIOUS LEARNING AND QUEST FOR PLEASURE

That is a phase of investigation and disclosure. You will continue through a phase of hyper consciousness to incredibly help reacquaint yourself together with your intuitive signs: hunger, season inclinations, and satiety.

This stage resembles figuring out how precisely to drive a vehicle. For the beginner driver, simply getting the vehicle out from the garage requires a lot of conscious deduction, loaded up with a psychological agenda: Place the principle component in the start, make certain the contraption is in diversion zone or impartial, start the motor, check the rearview reflect, remove the hand brake, and so forth. This hyper consciousness is basic to secure every one of the means required simply to acquire that vehicle into Drive! In a similar inclination, you will focus in on subtleties of eating which have advanced without such centred reasoning. (In any case, this is basic to recover the Intuitive Eater in you.)

It might seem clumsy and awkward, fanatical even. In any case, hyper consciousness varies than over the top considering. Over the top reasoning is generally unavoidable and is viewed as stress. It fills your brain during most of the day and prevents you from considering much else. Hyperconsciousness is increasingly specific. It zooms in the event that you have thought about food, yet leaves totally when the eating experience is finished. What's more, like the means required stresses become autopilot for the accomplished driver, Intuitive Eating will eventually get experienced without this fundamental ungainliness.

You may accept that you are in a hyperconscious state more often than not during this stage. This may feel awkward at first just as maybe even abnormal. Keep in mind, a ton of your prior eating was either primarily thoughtless or diet plan coordinated.

In this stage, you'll begin to make harmony with food giving yourself unqualified consent to expend. This part may feel frightening, and you may choose to move gradually (inside your solace level). Become acquainted with to wipe out blame incited eating and begin to find the requirement for the fulfilment component with food. The significantly progressively cheerful you are while expending, the substantially less you see food on the off chance that you are not hungry you won't wind up being lurking here and there. You will explore different avenues regarding foods that you probably won't have eaten for quite a while. This comprises of sifting through your exact food needs and needs. You may even find that you don't simply like the kind of a couple of the foods you've been longing for! (Remember those long stretches of dieting, or eating all that you "should" simply serve to disengage you from your own inner eating travel and genuine food decisions.) Become acquainted with to respect your food yearnings and perceive the body markers that show the innumerable degrees of appetite. Become acquainted with, to separate these organic pointers from the enthusiastic markers that may likewise trigger eating.

In this stage, you may find that you will eat bigger degrees of foods than the body needs. It will be difficult to regard your totality as of now since you will require time to try out the amount it requires to satisfy a denied sense of taste. What's more, it requires some serious energy that you ought to create trust with suppers again and comprehend that it's really okay to expend. By what means will you respect completion, on the off chance that you are not absolutely sure it's okay to eat the specific food, or if you fear it won't become there tomorrow?

In the event that you have recently been putting on overabundance weight, weight gain typically stops or is restricted to just a couple of pounds. At the point when you have been utilizing suppers inwardly, you may find that you will begin to feel your emotions and may encounter uneasiness, pity, or really sadness on occasion. Most of your eating could be foods that are heavier in fat and sugar than you've been familiar with in spite of the fact that you may have been eating huge degrees of these food types furtively or with blame. How you eat in this stage will never be the example that you'll set up or requirement for a lifetime. You will see that your nourishing soundness is for the most part helter-skelter and you probably won't feel physically alongside focuses during this time. That is all standard and anticipated. You have to let yourself continue through this phase for such a long time as you need. Keep in mind, and you are creating for quite a while of hardship, troublesome self-talk, and blame. You are re-building positive food experiences, much the same as a strand of pearls. Every feast experience, similar to each pearl, may seem immaterial, however, by and large, they change lives.

STAGE THREE: CRYSTALLIZATION

In this stage, you will experience the primary renewals of the Intuitive Eating style which has consistently been a piece of you, yet was covered underneath the flotsam and jetsam of dieting. At the point when you enter this stage, a great deal of the investigation work from the earlier stage begins to solidify and feels as if strong conducts change. Your thoughts regarding food are not any more over the top. You barely need to stay aware of the hyperconsciousness about eating that was initially required.

Thusly, your eating choices don't require very as particularly coordinated accepted. Rather, you find that your food choices and reactions to natural pointers are principally intuitive.

You have a bigger feeling of trust-both in your to pick what you really need to eat and in the undeniable reality that your natural signs are depend-capable. You are advantageous with your food choices and will start to see expanded satisfaction at your suppers. Now, you respect your appetite most of the time and it's less difficult to perceive what you feel simply like eating in the event that you are hungry. You keep on creating harmony with food.

What feels new in this stage is that it's more straightforward to require some investment out in the midst of your food to intentionally check exactly how a lot of your paunch is topping off. It is conceivable to watch your completion and regard the presence of that sign, regardless of whether you find that you as often as possible eat past the totality tag. Precisely like when a toxophilite requires focus on a crisp objective, it frequently requires catching numerous bolts before figuring out how precisely to come to the bull's-eye. You may at present be picking recently prohibited foods most of the time, yet you will find that you don't require as a lot of them to satisfy you.

On the off chance that you've been a genuinely signaled eater, you'll become very skilled at isolating natural yearning markers from passionate appetite. Because of this lucidity, more than not frequently, you'll be encountering your feelings and discovering techniques to com-stronghold and occupy yourself without the use of food.

Be certain you put weight decrease on the storage compartment burner. Much more significant than abundance weight reduction, is the inclination of well-turning out to be and strengthening that become-gins to happen. You won't any longer feel vulnerable and miserable. You will begin to regard your body and get that in case you're over your regular weight, it's because of the dieting attitude, rather than absence of resolve.

STAGE 4: THE INTUITIVE EATER AWAKENS

By enough time you arrive at this stage, all the work you have just been doing comes full circle in an agreeable, free-streaming eating style. You consistently pick what you truly need to eat when you are ravenous. Since you comprehend that you can have altogether more suppers, based on your personal preference, when you are starving, it's anything but difficult to stop eating when you are feeling serenely full. You may begin to find that you pick more advantageous foods, not on the grounds that you envision you should, but since you are feeling better physically when you take along these lines. The pressing need to demonstrate to yourself that you could have recently prohibited foods could have reduced. You truly know and trust these foods will be there, and on the off chance that you need to eat them truly, you can-in this manner they drop their charming quality. Chocolate starts to shield myself against a similar mental implication as a peach. You won't any more drawn out need to test yourself, just as your hardship reaction with suppers will be no more. At the point when you do choose the foods you used to limit, you'll get extraordinary delight, and feel content with a particularly littler amount than beforehand, and without blame. (At the point when you are feeling regretful eating a suppers, it removes a great deal of the happiness from eating.) In the event that managing your emotions have been hard for you, you'll be less reluctant to see them, and be increasingly capable at plunking down with them. Finding refreshing choices to occupy and comfort yourself when required can be normal for you. Your food talk and self talk will be certain and non-basic. Your tranquility settlement with suppers is solidly settled, and you will have discharged any contention or remaining blame about dinner's decisions you have hauled around. You have quit being furious together with your body and making ill bred input about it. You regard it and acknowledge there are a wide range of shapes and sizes on the planet. At this genuine point, and if it's intended to be, the body will be coming to moving toward its natural weight.

STAGE FIVE: THE ULTIMATE STAGE-TREASURE THE PLEASURE

Right now your Intuitive Eater has been guaranteed. You will confide in your body's intuitive capacities it will be easy to respect your yearning and regard totality. At long last, you will encounter no blame about your feast decisions or amounts. Since you like your sentimental relationship to dinners and fortune the fulfillment that eating currently offers you, you will dispose of unacceptable eating conditions and unappealing foods.

You should encounter benefiting from in the most ideal of conditions as opposed to corrupt it with enthusiastic misery. You will encounter an internal conviction to quit utilizing food to deal with enthusiastic circumstances, if that is your propensity. At the point when sentiments become too astounding, you will see that you'll much rather adapt to your feelings or occupy yourself at times from their site with anything separated from food.

Since your eating style has become a wellspring of joy rather than a suffering, you will encounter sustenance and development in various manners.

The duty of activity will be evacuated, and practicing will begin to look luring to you. Exercise won't be used as a driving strain to catch fire more calories; rather, you feel com-mitted to exercise with an end goal to feel much improved, and intellectually physically. In like manner, food won't be another instrument to make you feel terrible about how you eat; rather, it transforms into an approach to feeling as in reality great and solid as could be expected under the circumstances.

At the point when you arrive at a definitive stage, your bodyweight will sink into what's normal for you-a spot that is agreeable and befitting your height and body outline. In the event that your bodyweight was at that point ordinary, you will find that you'll keep up it without exertion and you will be freed of the mental good and bad times that go with the confinement/overeating cycles. Finally, you will encounter enabled and shielded from outside powers telling you what and exactly the amount to eat, and how the body should look. You will feel clear of the duty of dieting. What's more, you'll be an Intuitive Eater again.

THAT YOU CAN DO IT!

These stages and the progressions that happen with your eating and considerations may seem outlandish. Or on the other hand, it may show up excessively startling. For instance, the very idea of giving yourself unrestricted authorization to eat may seem unnerving and you may expect that you'll never stop eating or putting on abundance weight. The remainder of the distribution clarifies in extraordinary fine detail how precisely to execute every rule, why it truly is required, and the explanation behind it. Also, you will figure out how extra interminable dieters became Intuitive Eaters and how it changed their lives. By enough time you wrap up this book, you will unquestionably realize that you also may turn into an Intuitive Eater, and forestall the franticness of dieting.

CHAPTER 5:

GUIDELINE ONE: REJECT THE DIET MENTALITY

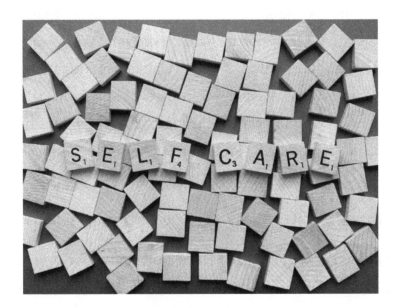

Eliminate diet books and magazine articles that give you false weight loss expectations quickly, effectively and forever. Get irate at the untruths which have driven you to feel like you were bombing each time a crisp diet plan quit working and you got back all the weight. If you permit really one little want to wait that a crisp and better diet might be prowling close by, it'll keep you from turning out to be clear to rediscover Intuitive Eating. In case you're similar to most of clients we see, the idea of not dieting could be startling (despite the fact that you comprehend that you can't force down one more diet program or drink). It's customary to encounter panicky about letting continue of dieting, especially when the globe around you is for the most part on some diet. It's been the main gadget you have perceived to lose pounds (yet incidentally). Winding up in a real predicament level is an incapacitating sense-doomed if you diet and accursed if you don't. A significant number of our clients feel caught between two clashing apprehensions: "Effectively keep dieting, I'll ruin my digestion and put on weight" and "Effectively quit dieting I'll put on increasingly overabundance weight." Other basic feelings of fear that individuals hear are:

FEAR: Easily quit dieting, I won't quit eating.

REALITY: Dieting is generally the outcome in for overeating. Of program it's difficult to abstain from eating when you've been under expending and confining dinners. It's a standard reaction to starvation (you'll discover increasingly about that inside the following section). However, when the body learns (and believes) that you'll not starve it anymore (through dieting), the outrageous drive for eating will diminish.

FEAR: I don't see how to eat when I'm not dieting.

REALITY: When you exile diet programs and be an Intuitive Eater, you'll be benefiting from because of inside signs, which may control your eating. That resembles figuring out how precisely to swim for the absolute first time. The sense to be encompassed by water could be frightening to the beginner swimmer, when completely submerged particularly. In like manner, being encompassed by dinners could be alarming to the ceaseless dieter, who's figuring out how precisely to eat once more. In any case, you'll not make sense of how to swim by just remaining at the upside of the pool (while accepting that figuring out how precisely to swim is an incredible thing). First you start by considering going all in and figuring out how to take in the water. In the end you will put your brain in the water in the event that you are prepared and you get helpful.

FEAR: I am out of control.

REALITY: Control is definitely not a worry in Intuitive Eating. Or maybe, you will rely on your inner signs, rather than on outside components and authority numbers (whom will undoubtedly challenge). No one might be the expert of "you." Just you know your thoughts, sentiments, and encounters. Become acquainted with to confide in your inward astuteness and can figure out how to focus on and respect your inside prompts (both physical and mental), which feels engaging.

THE DIET VOID

For some, a person dieting is an approach to deal with life, from topping off period, to filling in as representative of authority over your day by day life. Think about the changing occasions throughout your life where you began a diet plan. How as often as possible did your diet programs concur with troublesome events or changes in your everyday life? It's normal to begin a diet through the accompanying presence changes: moving from youth to youthfulness, going out, wedding, beginning a new activity, or while experiencing conjugal troubles. While dieting may have been worthless, it offered pleasure and expectation the elation of quick weight reduction and the invigoration of watching the level inch descending. The desire that this diet plan will work out; It's like prone to a hairdresser for a new trim, with the desire that it'll upset how you show up and feel about yourself and maybe completely changes you. Anyway when you state farewell to the fervor and joy of dieting, you'll likewise become letting continue of the bogus wish and dissatisfactions from dieting. There's a social segment to dieting that you may miss, diet plan holding. At the point when you decide to stop dieting, you might be astonished how often new diet plans and dieting will be the subjects of discourse at parties, with dear companions, at work-and right now you won't wind up being playing that game. It may feel simply like an absolute necessity see film numerous individuals are discussing, just you haven't saw it and furthermore have no plans to see it either. You may feel somewhat ignored, confined. Keep in mind, inasmuch as by and by there is money to be created; there will be a new contrivance or diet plan for a moment weight reduction fix. At one phase, the maker of something known as "Sleepers Dieter" asserted to incredibly assist individuals with achieving higher weight reduction during rest. Visit about dreaming! The producer was fined by the FTC to make unverified cases. Be that as it may, individuals still dished out the measure of cash on account of this new trick.

THE ONE-LAST-DIET TRAP

Stage one to turning into an Intuitive Eater is to dismiss the dietary plan attitude. However despite the fact that you come to conditions with the vanity and harm that dieting releases on your body (and brain), it's somewhat a troublesome initially rung on the stepping stool. To get yourself out from the last-chance diet plan trap, you need to come to conditions with the established truth that dieting doesn't work and can, really, be unsafe. (Remember, an assortment of study shows that the make a move of dieting raises your risk of putting on much more weight. This is valid for children, young people, and grown-ups. We imagine that if individuals really realized that starting a better eating routine could make the body put on increasingly abundance weight, they would not so much decline the vain dieting course.) Maybe you're slanted to contend, be that as it may, that you'll encounter better about yourself when you lose the abundance weight. Yet, thinks about have shown that enhancements in mental prosperity associated with weight reduction are basically as present moment as the pounds dropped and recovered. The "extraordinary feelings" decrease with recaptured pounds, and existing issues of self-well worth and general passionate capacity return to introductory sums when the overabundance weight is recovered.

PSEUDO-DIETING

Many customers state, "I've deserted dieting" anyway despite everything they have issues shaking the dietary plan mindset. They may be physically from a diet, anyway the dieting contemplations remain. The issue is normally that dieting contemplations for the most part bring about diet-like practices, which transforms into pseudo-dieting or oblivious dieting. Therefore, these clients will even now endure the average reactions of dieting, yet it's especially harder to distinguish (and they truly feel wild with their eating). Pseudo-dieting practices aren't normally clear to the individual occupied with them. Recollect that eating is surely basic that it's difficult to get objective. It could be hard to procure the escape clauses inside your own expending mindset/conduct if you don't know very well what you are scanning for. To the stun of our clients they customarily don't find that they have just been pseudo-dieting until on the whole we assess their Intuitive Eating diary. Here are a couple of instances of pseudo-dieting:

a. Meticulously checking starch grams might be the cutting edge version of tallying calories. While monitoring what you eat offers its merits, the demonstration of tallying sugar grams to control weight is quite not quite the same as checking calories. Many ceaseless dieters are benefits at apportioning their sugar grams for the afternoon and they are caught.

b. Eating just "free from any potential harm" foods. This outcome in staying with sans fat of charge as well as low-calorie foods, wind up being-yond tallying starch grams. For example, one customer wouldn't regularly eat any dinners that recorded a few gram of muscle to fat ratio on the supper's name, whatever her all out muscle versus fat and calorie utilization for your day was. Keep in mind, in any case, that one suppers, one feast, or 1 day won't represent the deciding moment your prosperity or your weight.

c. Eating just now and again of the day, regardless of whether you are hungry, is normally a typical extra propensity from dieting, particularly not eating following a specific time of night, such as after 6 P.M. Rude awakening: Our life structures don't punch period timekeepers; we don't all of a sudden mood killer our requirement for vitality at a particular time. This can particularly be viewed as an issue for a dieter who practices after work, returns late around 7:30 P.M., and chooses it's also late to expend for fear that the overabundance fat meter is certainly in high apparatus. In spite of the fact that it is sensible never to need to visit bed on a total stomach since it will be terrible, to deny a destitute body any dinners or vitality can be outlandish.

d. Paying compensation for eating "poor" foods such as treats, cheesecake, or frozen yogurt. The punishment run from avoiding another feast, eating less, vowing to become "extraordinary" tomorrow, or performing additional activity.

e. Reducing on food, especially when feeling fat or at whatever point an uncommon occasion like a wedding or course get-together comes up. While diminishing sounds guiltless a lot of, it's astounding how as often as possible this gets carried on in the kind of oblivious under eating. Keep in mind, under eating for the most part triggers overeating.

f. Pacifying food desires by drinking coffee or diet pop. That is a typical dieting procedure to mitigate food longings without eating or calorie utilization.

g. Limiting starches. We are struck by the measure of clients who proclaim they comprehend of the requirement for eating this sort of fuel, anyway eat an insufficient amount of starches, such as breads, pasta, rice, and so forth, since they're apprehensive they will put on weight.

h. Gaining a "bogus food experience" in open zones. You just eat what's "appropriate" before others. One client, Alice, ate a fantastic dinner with companions. At the point when the sweet plate landed around her really needed a touch of pie, yet battled the longing, since she wished to resemble the sound/weight-careful eater. For any case, on her benefit way home, the longing for the pie expand into a wild hankering. Alice ended at the shop, purchased a total pie, and ate one-fourth of it- much more than she'd have eaten experienced she respected her precise food inclination! This relational dieting conduct of increasing a bogus food experience exploded backward (and it much of the time does).

i. Competing with someone else who's dieting ... feeling committed to wind up being similarly high-minded (or significantly more). Since dieting can be viewed as an ethical characteristic inside our general public, it isn't bizarre that you'll get sucked into appearing temperate. This can just happen when companions, family, or a considerable other is dieting.

j. Second-speculating or judging all that you have the right to expend predicated on what you've eated promptly in the day, rather than on hunger signs. One client, Sally, ate two colossal dishes of puffed rice oat for breakfast subsequent to working for 60 minutes. She accepted that was an exorbitant measure of food and later on in the midmorning didn't enable herself to expend, in spite of the fact that she was voracious. Sally figured, "How may I be hungry only two hours when I had an enormous breakfast?" reality for Sally was that while her degree of food every morning was greater than her standard, it had been as yet deficient for the amount of activity she did. Her body was endeavoring to advise her, "I need more fuel." However Sally felt regretful to be ravenous. She additionally felt remorseful for eating an enormous breakfast, until she perceived that much of the time she had under eaten. Wish dinner or tidbit won't fit the "standard" part size from your very own dieting days; it by and large doesn't infer you are overeating!

k. Learning to be a veggie lover or expending a gluten gratis diet restricted to the reason for thinning down. A veggie lover way of life could be a sound method for expending and living, however on the off chance that it's grasped with a diet plan attitude; it turns out to be essentially another diet. For instance, Karen began eating meatless to lose overabundance weight. In any case, every month into her veggie lover eating, she began wanting meat. Nothing you've seen earlier had she encountered meats longings!

Karen saw she barely ever truly planned to transform into a veggie lover. She wasn't contemplating veggie lover eating for health or moral issues, similarly as a vehicle to get more fit, in this manner her diet back once more terminated.

THE DIETER'S DILEMMA

Regardless of whether you are occupied with genuine dieting or pseudo-dieting, any sort of dieting will prompt confusions. The acquire vanity of dieting is typically depicted in the Dieter's Problem outline delivered by clinicians, John P. G and foreyt. Ken Goodrick, showed underneath. The Dieter's Problem is normally activated by the need to be slender, that prompts dieting. That is the point at which the issue unfurls. Dieting raises longings and desires for dinners. The dieter yield to the hankering, gorges, lastly recovers any lost overabundance weight. He's back again to where he started, with the underlying weight-or higher. When again the dieter persuades the need to be slim ... thusly another diet starts. The Dieter's Dilemma is certainly sustained and deteriorates with each difference in the everyday practice. The dieter can be heavier and feels much increasingly wild with eating.

INSTRUCTIONS TO REJECT THE DIETARY PLAN MENTALITY

To disregard the dieting legend and the dieting mindset, our contemplations require another system of reference. In the top of the line distribution, The 7 Habits of Effective People, essayist Stephen Covey advanced the possibility of perspective changes. A worldview is positively a model or collection of reference where we see and comprehend the world. In the superb universe of weight the executives, dieting might be the social worldview where we attempt to control our pounds. A change in outlook is regularly a break with custom, with old methods for deduction, with matured ideal models. We should change our worldview to dismiss dieting; simply after that would we be able to make a solid sentimental association with dinners and our bodies.

While Covey's capacity is focused at the business network, he hits upon a worry that groups valid for interminable dieters. He accepts that people are much of the time attracted to treatment the issue without regard to the long haul ramifications of the "handy solution." He feels that this methodology really intensifies the issue rather than for all time understanding it. He factors to the physical body as a prized resource that every now and again is typically destroyed while one is for the most part on the challenge for quick results and momentary advantages. Recorded underneath are the means to begin your change in perspective of dismissing the dietary plan mindset.

STAGE ONE: RECOGNIZE AND ACKNOWLEDGE THE HARM THAT DIETING CAUSES

There exists a generous measure of learn about the damage that dieting causes. Recognize that the harm is genuine, and that kept dieting is just going to propagate your issues. A couple of the key undesirable impacts gathered from fundamental examinations are clarified beneath in two gatherings, enthusiastic and natural. As you read, have an individual stock, and have yourself which of the issues you as of now are encountering. Perceiving that dieting might be the issue can assist you with getting through the social fantasy that diets work. Keep in mind; if dieting might be the issue, how might it take part the solution?

DAMAGE FROM DIETING: BIOLOGICAL AND HEALTH

Atlanta separate from lawyers century, starvation and human starvation have existed. Tragically, this is genuine at the present time. Natural selection recently structured endurance of the fattest-just individuals that have adequate vitality stores (abundance fat) could endure a starvation. Subsequently, our life structures are as yet equipped in this present day to battle starvation at the cell level.

So far as the body can be included, dieting is a sort of starvation (regardless of the way that it's deliberate).

a. Chronic dieting encourages your body to hold more fat when you start eating once more. Low-calorie diets double the chemicals that produce and store fat in your body. This is a sort of organic remuneration to enable the body to store more vitality, or additional fat, subsequent to dieting.

b. Chronic dieting eases back the rate of weight loss with each progressive attempt to diet. It has been exhibited in both rodent and person contemplates.

c. Decrease digestion. Dieting triggers your body to turn out to be better at using calorie utilization by diminishing the body's reliance on vitality.

d. Boost gorges and yearnings. The two people and rodents have been demonstrated to indulge after constant food limitation. Food limitation invigorates the psyche to discharge a course of longings to expend more. After generous overabundance weight reduction, thinks about likewise show that rodents pick expending progressively fat, while people have been appeared to pick foods both immersed in fat and sugar.

e. Increase risk of untimely death toll and heart disease. A thirty-two-year study more prominent than 3,000 ladies and men in the Framingham Center Study has exhibited that regardless of starting pounds, individuals whose fat more than once rises and down-known as overabundance weight cycling or yo-yo dieting-have an expanded by and large demise check and double the standard danger of kicking the bucket of cardiovascular ailment. These outcomes had been free of cardiovascular hazard factors, and remained constant whether an individual was thin or hefty. The damage from yo-yo dieting may be equivalent to the dangers of remaining corpulent.

Correspondingly, results of the Harvard Alumni Health Study show that people who lose and gain at any rate eleven pounds inside ten years or somewhere in the vicinity, don't live inasmuch as the individuals who keep up a very much adjusted weight.

f. Trigger satiety prompts to decay. Dieters for the most part quit eating because of a deliberate point of confinement rather than internal signs of totality. This, combined with skip-ping foods, can condition you to expend suppers of progressively greater size.

g. Trigger body shape to change. Yo-yo dieters who consistently recapture the lost pounds will in general recover fat in the stomach region. This sort of fat stockpiling heightens the danger of cardiovascular illness.

Other written undesirable impacts incorporate cerebral pains, menstrual anomalies, exhaustion, dried out skin, and hair diminishing.

DAMAGE FROM DIETING: PSYCHOLOGICAL AND EMOTIONAL

Mental experts announced the following advertisement section impacts at the milestone 1992 National Institutes of Health, Excess weight reduction and Control Conference:

a. Dieting is related with eating issue. (Inside a disconnected research, dieters were eight events as prone to have issues with a benefiting from scatter by age fifteen, than non-dieters.)

b. Dieting could make pressure or help make the dieter progressively defenseless to its belongings. Autonomous of bodyweight itself, dieting is generally associated with feelings of fizzling, brought down confidence, and relational nervousness.

c. The dieter is much of the time helpless against decrease of control overeating while disregarding "the rules" of the dietary plan, regardless of whether there was a real or saw offense of the dietary plan. The unimportant view of expending a taboo suppers (independent of real calorie content) will do to bring about overeating. In another report, analysts David Garner and Susan

Wooley present a convincing defense against the significant expense of bogus wish from dieting. They infer that:

d. Dieting consistently dissolves certainty and individual trust.

e. Many obese individuals expect they can't have become corpulent except if they had some basic character deficiency. Garner and Wooley contend that despite the fact that numerous corpulent individuals may encounter gorging and sadness, these psychological and social manifestations will be the aftereffect of dieting. Be that as it may, these overweight individuals effectively translate these indications as extra verification a basic issue. However, large individuals don't have extreme enthusiastic unsettling influences in contrast with ordinary weight individuals.

STAGE 2: BE FAMILIAR WITH DIET MENTALITY CHARACTERISTICS AND THINKING

The diet attitude regions in unobtrusive structures, despite the fact that you decide to dismiss dieting. It's fundamental that you perceive basic highlights of the dietary plan attitude; it will illuminate you on the off chance that you are as yet playing the dieting computer game. Disregard self discipline, getting respectful, and coming up short.

The general attributes of the way the dieter versus the non-dieter see eating, exercise, and improvement are outlined by a diagram beneath:

DISREGARD WILLPOWER.

While just no specialist would anticipate that an individual should "will" blood flow strain to ordinary levels, specialists much of the time anticipate that their overweight individual should "will" their weight reduction by confining their food, as per Susan Z. Yanovski, M.D. That is additionally a predominant disposition among our clients and numerous Americans-all you will require is generally resolution and only a little restraint. In a 1993 Gallup Poll, the most run of the mill obstruction referred to thinning somewhere around women was determination.

For example, Marilyn is an amazingly fruitful lawyer who moved to the absolute best of the association stepping stool. She acknowledges her accomplishment for her commitment, resolve, and self-control. Be that as it may, when she endeavored to utilize these model ideas in her dieting endeavors, she bombed consistently. Whatever accomplishment she had achieved in her expert presence was dulled by her sentiment of coming up short with her eating.

For what reason was Marilyn in a situation to be in this manner taught in a solitary zone of her reality be that as it may, not in the extra? "Self-discipline" gets from the term follower. Identifying with Stephen Covey's work, on the off chance that you are a follower to your own profound qualities which have a superseding design, all things considered, you'll have the will to move them out. Marilyn thought profoundly that creating demanding understandings and keeping perfect data had been necessities to building self-assurance with her clients and her legal counselor. In any case, some way or another, hearing that bread wasn't right utilizing one diet plan and anything with sugars was off base on another, didn't incite a similar kind of profound convictions. Attempt as she may, she couldn't generally feel that chocolate chip treats had been that insidious!

Self control can be disclosed as a push to counter characteristic wishes and supplant them with proscriptive rules. It additionally suggests the ability to do terrible employments that aren't basic.

The longing to have desserts is common, standard, and very agreeable! Any diet that tells you that you can't have desserts is absolutely conflicting with your natural want. The dietary plan be-comes a few inflexible rules, and these sorts of rules can just barely trigger insubordination.

Self control won't have a place in Intuitive Feeding on. As Marilyn turned into an Intuitive Eater, she found that meeting her own pointers fortified her natural senses, than countering them rather. She had no one else's proscriptive standards to follow or to oppose. Marilyn has stopped battling the ghost self discipline battle and has delivered harmony with suppers and her body.

DISREGARD BEING OBEDIENT

A good natured recommendation by a life partner or life partner such as: "Honey, you should have the seared chicken... "Or "You shouldn't eat those fries... ", can set off an inward food resistance. In this sort of food battle, your only weapons store to battle turns into a twofold order of fries. We call this "overlooks you eating."

In material science, opposition consistently happens as a response to constrain. We see this hypothesis doing his thing in the public eye revolts as often as possible emits when the weight of power becomes also incredible. Likewise, the simple demonstration to be advised how to continue (really if it's something you ought to do), can bring about a defiant chain reaction. Precisely like "horrible two-year-olds" or teenagers who revolt to show they are autonomous, dieters can start defiant eating in light of the make a move of dieting, utilizing its gathering of unbending standards.

In this way, it's not stunning to tune in to from our clients that breaking the rules of a diet plan make them feel like they did on the off chance that they were rebellious youngsters. Yet, take focus, resistance is a standard work of self-protection shielding your space, or individual limits. Think about an individual limit as a high block fence encompassing you, with just 1 entryway. Just you can open up that entryway, if you pick. Thusly, no one is permitted inside, except if you welcome the person in. Inside your fence dwell individual feelings, musings, and organic pointers. People who expect they comprehend the thing you require and advise you how to continue are choosing the lock to your door, or attacking your limits. Keep in mind; no one might be the expert of "you." Just you know your thoughts, emotions, and encounters. No one might comprehend what's inside, except if he is told by you, by welcoming him in. What diet or diet plan advocate may potentially know whether you are starving or exactly what amount of food it will require to fulfill you? How would anybody yet you know very well what surface and flavor sensations will get satisfying to your sense of taste? In the brilliant universe of dieting, individual limits are crossed at numerous sums. For example, you are determined what things to eat, exactly its amount to expend, and when to eat it. These choices should all wind up being close to home decisions, with deference for explicit self-rule and body markers. While food direction will originate from somewhere else, you ought to in the long run be responsible for the when, what, and exactly the amount of eating.

DISREGARD FAILURE.

Our incessant dieters head into our workplaces feeling just as they are disappointments. Regardless of whether they are profoundly situated administrators, conspicuous whizzes, or straight-An understudy, every one of them talk about their food experiences despicably, and they question whether they'll ever be able to feel effective in the area of eating. The dietary plan attitude strengthens feelings of progress or coming up short. You can't fall flat at Intuitive Eating-it's a learning strategy at each point in transit. What used to become viewed as a mishap will rather be viewed as an ascent experience. You'll get back progressing nicely when you watch this as progress, not disappointment.

Stage 3: Eliminate The Dieter's Tools

The dieter relies upon outer powers to adjust his eating, staying with a controlled diet, eating since now is the ideal time, or eating just a predetermined (and estimated) sum, regardless of whether hungry or not. The dieter additionally approves progress by outside powers, the scale principally, asking, "Exactly what number of pounds have I lost?" "Is my abundance weight up or down?" It is period to dispose of your dieting devices. Dispose of the feast programs and the suppers and restroom scales.

On the off chance that all it required was a magnificent "reasonable" calorie-confined dinner expect to shed pounds, we'd be viewed as a country of thin human free feast plans are ample from magazines, papers, the Internet, and even some food organizations.

STAGE 4: BECOME COMPASSIONATE TOWARD YOURSELF

At the point when the world about you is dieting, and euphoric about how precisely weight is dissolving off subsequently of the most recent diet plan fever it's reasonable that you could get pulled in. Be that as it may, this draw is generally significantly something beyond style. In her distribution, The Religion of Thinness, Harvard-prepared scholar and researcher, Michelle M. Lelwica makes a convincing contention about how precisely the unending mission for slenderness, through dieting, satisfies an otherworldly food desires. The journey for dieting goes about as a "biggest reason" by:

a. Providing two or three fantasies to accept about the "benefits" of slimness.
b. Giving ceremonies to organize the everyday lives of women.
c. Creating an ethical code which to live and eat by.
d. Creating a typical relationship and a network for females.

Considering these secret "benefits" of dieting, just no big surprise you may get tempted by the "benefits" of dieting. Try not to overcome yourself okay with intriguing dreams of attempting one more diet or simply endeavoring to diet. It requires some investment to disregard this craving, despite the fact that you mentally under-stand that the journey for dieting is really vain.

ADAPT TOGETHER TO YOUR EMOTIONS WITHOUT REQUIRING FOOD

Discover approaches to solace and straightforwardness, support, divert, and fathom your issues without requiring food. Stress, forlornness, fatigue, and outrage are sentiments the greater part of us experience all through presence. Everyone has its trigger and every offer its very own mollification. Suppers won't fix these sentiments. It could comfort for the present moment, divert from the uneasiness, or really numb you directly into a food headache. Be that as it may, food won't resolve the issue.

On the off chance that anything, eating for a passionate craving is just going to make you feel more terrible after some time. You'll in the long run need to adapt to the wellspring of the feeling, alongside the distress of overeating.

Benefiting from doesn't happen in a void. Of your weight in any case, food generally has mental affiliations. In the event that you have any uncertainty, catch a look at supper's advertisements. They drive our eating catches not so much through our stomachs yet through the mental association. They suggest in sixty negligible seconds or less you may:

a. Capture sentiment with a sentimental mug of espresso/coffee
b. Bake somebody glad.
c. Incentive yourself with an affluent treat.

Eating can be one of the most genuinely loaded experiences that we have in our lives. The mental mood to expending is characterized from the principal day time that the newborn child develops the bosoms or the container to suppress his crying. It's at that point fortified at whatever points a treat rises to relieve a scratched knee, or frozen yogurt is normally eaten to celebrate only a youth baseball triumph. Almost every culture and religion utilizes food as a fundamental representative custom, from the American Thanksgiving blowout to the Jewish Passover Seder. At whatever point a critical life experience is praised with dinners, the mental association develops, from the I-got-the-advancement-ner extraordinary occasion to the yearly birthday cake. Moreover, each time food is used for a little twisted licking or solace, the enthusiastic relationship reinforces.

Food is love, dinners are comfort, suppers are prize, and dinners are a confided in companion. What's more, some of the time, food turns into your solitary companion in events of agony and dejection. The eating experience itself, overeating particularly, inspires sentiments, and the ones emotions have any kind of effect your ability to eat typically. Likely the most hindering feelings that overeating can stir up are blame and disgrace. Studies have exhibited that in spite of the fact that you may have prompt passionate solace from eating, the negative rush of blame that blasts forward is ground-breaking a lot of to totally dispose of the alleviation.

If you supplant the blame with feelings of self-sympathy, you'll become liberated to concentrate on your basic issues and discover techniques to get them and adapt to them.

Getting an Intuitive Eater implies seeing how to wind up being delicate with yourself about how precisely you use dinners to arrangement, and letting continue of the blame. As odd as this would sound, eating may have been the simply way of dealing with stress you'd to finish troublesome events in your day by day life. It might in like manner have been an unavoidable outcome of long periods of dieting and feelings of hardship and gloom that emerged from dieting. Dieting itself can bring about feelings, which at last outcome in utilizing food to deal with these sentiments chalks up another horrible everyday practice because of dieting.

THE CONTINUUM OF EMOTIONAL EATING

Food can be used to deal with sentiments in a variety of ways. Utilizing food as such isn't a component of organic appetite, however of passionate food yearnings. Enthusiastic eating is unquestionably activated by emotions, such as weariness or outrage, not by food desires. These sentiments can bring about anything from a kind snack to a crazy gorge. It's fundamental that you perceive that this adapting framework lies on a continuum of solidarity that starts toward one side with moderate, practically general tactile expending despite what might be expected end with desensitizing, anesthetizing eating regularly.

RAISING AN INTUITIVE EATER: WHAT WORKS TOGETHER WITH KIDS AND TEENS

We will in general be inquired as to whether it's conceivable to train youngsters Intuitive Eating. The appropriate response isn't simply can you truly assist youngsters with returning to the Intuitive Eaters these were during childbirth, in any case it is frequently less troublesome than with grown-ups. Kids are significantly less questionable than grown-ups and much increasingly open and anxious. How about we start with avoidance. At the point when a kid is conceived, this kid has the inborn capacity had a need to see how to eat.

I was fortunately enough as of late to go to a companion's little girl, who had essentially conceived an offspring fourteen days before to her wonderful child young lady. Alexis was just getting increasingly alright with the staggering errand of deciding what to look like after her new conceived. Which cry planned that she was lethargic, which said that there is a diaper that necessary changing, and which let her comprehend that the infant had a need to eat? Presently, in the event that you've at any point watched a destitute child; you comprehend that her most unmistakable cry might be the one of food longings. On the off chance that the child is neglected when she's ravenous, she'll shout and shout until gave the bosoms or jug.

The yearning signal is intensely intended for about all infants, and there exists a characteristic nature to help make the reliance on sustenance known. I was situated and talking with Alexis, when little Lily made the sounds that let her mother comprehend that she was starving. To sit watching this dazzling association among mother and kid was a real blessing. Lily breast fed utilizing one bosom and the other, so when she was finished, she dismissed her important head and nodded off. Alexis was in amazement of how intuitive her newborn child's eating experience was.

In the event that there is attunement to the wide cluster of obvious and nuanced messages that the kid offers, the child will grow up with a sentiment of self-self-assurance that his needs work and will be normally met. At the point when the child is hungry and is typically immediately encouraged, numerous significant correspondences will become passed on. The first message is that food desires is an all regular, ordinary, and "right" sensation. Later on, the impression of food desires will be related to the movement to discover food. An adjusted reaction to the kid's food longings will evoke a sentiment of security, taking out any worry with hardship. In the event that, rather, this essential need of the youngster isn't met at the right occasions, the kid will begin to expect that there won't be sufficient food. Accordingly, this child is in danger of quieting hunger signals, rather than believing that the food desires signal is a confided in message all through life. Envision a newborn child whose set on an encouraging everyday practice, a thing that was a typical proposal from ages later. The mother or father was encouraged to put the newborn child on an everyday practice of eating, which go from each 2-3 hours to each 3 to 4 hours. Numerous guardians reacted emphatically to the proposal, as managing the eating plan enables them to plan throughout the day consistently ahead of time. Of program, most guardians didn't receive this system out of egotistical requires. These were advised a customary sustaining timetable will be best for the child. Lamentably, this is basically not for the most part the situation, as this technique gets the possibility to make various issues. On the off chance that the child got starving and cried around 30 minutes before the booked time, the mother or father was provoked to keep down to sustain her. Assuming, be that as it may, the child wasn't yet starving right now, she might be cajoled to eat at any rate. Since craving and completion signals were not normally being strengthened, the destitute, shouting child or the not so much yet starving infant was on his strategy to doubting these powerful messages. For the destitute baby, the potential worry with future hardship may flourish. For the infant who was propelled to eat before food desires had adequately shown up, false impressions and protection from benefiting from can develop. For a youngster who was basically benefited from plan, than on request somewhat, moving to the baby years can start a confused sentimental association with food. On the off chance that a decent measure of food gets open to a youngster who encountered a feeling of hardship earliest stages, the kid could be inclined to build up a characteristic propensity to indulge. At the point when another feast is offered, 1 of 2 potential outcomes may happen. The youngster might just be excessively finished and won't eat or may surpass this totality transmission and take in much more suppers, amassing for another potential starvation. For the child who was just persuaded to expend as a newborn child, the opportunity to eat much more autonomously as a baby may likewise introduce two potential outcomes. He may proceed relentlessly to expend when he's not yet starving, or he could apply his autonomy by declining to eat.

Luckily, today encouraging calendars are once in a while prescribed, and upright parental figures tend to react habitually to the youngster's appetite signals. Be that as it may, shouldn't something be said about signs totality? Have you at any point truly attempted to keep to encourage a youngster after she dismisses her psyche from the bosoms or jug, since you're terrified that she lacks sustenance or that she's not so much developing rapidly a lot of? At the point when that youngster's belly is unquestionably full, she will typically recoil from turning out to be coercively fed. We've seen, with loathsomeness, little children who were oftentimes convinced to eat much more than they required, all through their underlying couple of years.

At last they either put on significantly more abundance weight than was empowering or wound up participating in dinners battles and would not expend particularly by any stretch of the imagination. For example, the mother of an amazingly youthful customer was in certainty portrayed youngster defensive arrangements by the specialist stirred up in treatment. This mother had procured a sister who experienced died in a starved condition from anorexia nervosa. Because of this, she related getting underweight with death toll and became alarmed that her child will be underweight. As an all out outcome, she stuffed her little kid with enormous quantities of food. This is seen as enthusiastic kid misuse.

The most essential piece of guaranteeing that a child holds the greater part of his intrinsic capacity around craving and completion is trust. Ellyn Satter, in her weighty book, Child of Mine: Feeding with Like and Good Sense (2000), relevantly says that it's the guardians' business to supply the dinners, and the youngster's work to expend to such an extent or short of what he prerequisites. In early stages, it's occasional a parent veers off out of this give and consider, however as youngsters re-situate of the "milk simply" arrange, guardians have an undeniably increasingly troublesome period staying tuned legitimately into a kid's eating markers. Guardians believe that there are along these lines many "authentic" known explanations behind them to endeavor to deal with the kid's expending. In this time of the plague of youth weight issues, the fear of a child putting on an inordinate measure of weight regularly prospects good natured pediatricians to give guardians the direction to watch what and how especially a child is eating.

The contrary circumstance may likewise be available, when there is a fear that the child isn't putting on enough weight. Moreover, numerous guardians who wish to enable their children to be as solid since they can empower them to eat just healthfully dense foods and restrict them from play suppers. In spite of the fact that this attempt to control the aggregate sum and sort of food kids are eating is regularly conceived from extraordinary goals, what's more, it brings the possibility of the child's question of his signs. Not just are his food longings and completion markers missed, yet additionally his intrinsic under-standing up of his food decisions and how his body appears to be subsequent to eating various amounts and sorts of food sources. As opposed to hearing and regarding her own physical responses to the eating experience, the child responds to the mother or father's outer message, rather than her very own inner comprehension. This response can have immense varieties to be the "acceptable little woman" and performing everything that Mommy wants, to performing out as the insubordinate child, who won't eat most, everything.

THE SCIENCE AND PSYCHOLOGY OF INTUITIVE EATING

Imagine a reality where you woke up every day and had a basic association with food. You ate when you were hungry and stopped when you were full. There are no events other than a picnic for you. Do not be defeated when you have eaten something "terrible". There is simply no shame or guilt. Don't eat out of anger or misery. You just ate what felt solid and your body. In spite of prevalent thinking, this isn't a story book.

This sort of association with dinners is most likely conceivable. Suppose you realized that you had a need to do to get it going was to trust - trust the body and you to at last make educated alternatives encompassing food?

Trust is the middle purpose of a dietary way of thinking alluded to as Intuitive Taking in. It's by creating depending upon your body's interior signs in regards to food yearnings and totality that you could start to make extraordinary decisions around eating. You can recognize physical and mental yearnings and over the long haul you'll see that you could eat in a way that enables you to find your characteristic abundance weight and health. This methodology is clearly not equivalent to what we typically hear. No more does great medical coverage and regular pounds require diet programs, calorie limitation, and exceptional exercise. A remarkable opposite, the simple demonstration of hearing the body, believing its insight and respecting its prerequisites can bring about weight decrease, improved vitality and a greatly improved encounter of life. In case you're keen on this methodology, recorded beneath are 4 significant bits of knowledge in to the science and the brain research of Intuitive Eating and exactly why it truly works:

THERE IS A BRAIN IN YOUR BELLY

The information behind eating intuitively is in truth situated in science. Have you at any point persevered through a "feeling" that something had not been correct? Maybe you have felt "off" utilizing conditions? Felt butterflies in your paunch? Or on the other hand encountered an annoyed mid-region when needing to deal with a situation you encountered uncertain about? That is your bodies enteric on edge framework talking, generally alluded to as the "gut-mind." Yes, we do have a brain inside our tummy. Our "gut-brain," of program, contrasts from the brain in our psyche. The enteric apprehensive program is really housed underneath the mucosal covering and between your strong layers of the throat, the stomach, and the little and internal organs. Through an extraordinarily complex system of neurons and neuro-synthetic compounds; authorizes and controls events in different regions of the body, similar to the brain itself. Specialists have confirmed that the enteric sensory system is consistently giving data to your minds in regards to our dietary necessities. The greater part of us make sense of how to eat by hearing messages originating from past ourselves - correspondences from our folks, educators, companions, or the press. Eating intuitively needs respecting the messages from your internal method to acquire knowing to support you.

YOUR BODY COMPREHENDS WHEN IT'S HUNGRY AND WHEN IT TRULY IS FULL.

Starting the technique of seeing how to trust your "gut-mind" and your body framework shrewdness implies understanding your body's internal signs concerning yearning and completion. It's imperative to such an extent that you decelerate and watch with the goal that you can hear what the body is stating. Periodically, we're moving in this manner rapidly through the globe that individuals spend our period separated from the body. We run in one gathering to another, skip suppers at whatever point we don't have period, or indulge before a day's over. This separation unleashes destruction on our pace of digestion and on our euphoria. On the off chance that you begin to tune into the body, you'll perceive what it feels as if when you're hungry and full. Your body will tell you when you're exhausted or vigorous or experiencing issues processing. Watch your body's messages. How would you experience when you're ravenous? Will your stomach experience light and rumble? Do you get yourself slight cerebral pains or does the mouth territory start to water? Notice on the off chance that you are starting to feel full. Where do you feeling it inside your body? In your belly? Do you start to unwind or inhale less troublesome? Everybody is extraordinary; subsequently we'll all have our own special real sensations and instant messages. You have to time to ask the body what it needs. Check out the vibes of food desires and totality and you'll be en route to eating intuitively.

BELIEVING THE BODY BENEFITS YOUR HEALTH FROM MULTIPLE WAYS

Probably the greatest blessing you may get from benefiting from intuitively is the capacity to confide in both the body and yourself. This may have significant advantages without anyone else generally speaking health. Obviously, everybody comprehends that pressure is hard for our health. Washing ourselves in strain hormones consistently makes it hard to lose overabundance weight and assemble muscle. It can cause depletion and debilitate invulnerability. Be that as it may, believing your body's inward prompts and feeling guaranteed in this methodology empowers you to loosen up into your sentimental association with food in addition to your reality. Envision the stream straight down impact this may have without anyone else generally speaking admirably turning out to be. Trusting and getting the expert on yourself just as your very own needs can make you are feeling progressively engaged to cause an actual existence where you too can truly flourish.

By putting trust in yourself you may start to feel more secure in your connections and on the planet. You may find that you can move away from being no picnic for yourself to being increasingly caring. From that point, self-judgment around food can turn into a relic of past times. Kindly don't disparage the intensity of setting trust in your body and yourself.

HEALTH AND WELL-BEING

Positive health brain science speaks to the requests subterranean insect end of enthusiastic states, which incorporate inclination perky, glad, thankful, and has been appeared by a few examinations to foresee future degrees of health and prosperity. In addition, these impacts amass and compound after some time, making individuals more beneficial, all the more socially coordinated, powerful, and versatile. Additionally, there are reported physical medical advantages of such states, which incorporate lower levels of the pressure chemical cortisol and less aggravation. An investigation by Tylka and Wilcox (2006) on 340 school ladies demonstrated that two center develops of Intuitive Eating, (1) eating for physical instead of passionate reasons and (2) dependence on inner craving and satiety signals to decide when and the amount to eat, exceptionally adds to the mental prosperity including: idealism, mental solidness (a pointer of strength, or the capacity to recoup from affliction), genuine self-respect, beneficial outcome, proactive adapting, and social critical thinking.

The examination's discoveries feature the significance of an individual's capacity to identify and take care of their feelings and their organic prompts of craving and satiety, as location and consciousness of these states are particularly associated with prosperity. These discoveries approve a significant number of the Intuitive Eating standards (Honor Your Hunger, Respect Your Fullness, Coping with Feelings without Using Food, Reject the Diet Mentality).

INTUITIVE EATING HOLDS PROMISE FOR U.S. MILITARY

The U.S. Armed force led a promising pilot study on the benefits of Intuitive Eating for its soldiers (Heilson and Cole 2011). Analysts from the U.S. Armed force Baylor graduate program in sustenance assessed both inspirations for eating and the Intuitive Eating qualities of one hundred dynamic obligation military assistance individuals matured eighteen to sixty-five years of age. The outcomes showed that military assistance individuals with an ordinary weight file scored the most noteworthy on the Intuitive Eating Scale, were bound to eat for physical reasons, and depended upon their inner craving satiety signs, while members with better than average weight record levels were slanted to eat for non-intuitive or nonphysical reasons. In view of these promising outcomes, a bigger report is in progress, which will assess the viability of an Intuitive Eating system to help break the enthusiastic, ecological, and social association with eating in the military assistance.

SELF-SILENCING

Self-silencing is the concealment of one's contemplations, emotions, or necessities and it is a sexual orientation marvel affecting ladies' psychological wellness. The procedure of self-quieting is thought to start in youthfulness, a defenseless time when body disappointment and social weights develop. While quieting their voices, young ladies may start to disregard or smother physiological or hunger signals that are conflicting with cultural thoughts of slenderness. Articulation of considerations, emotions, or necessities seems, by all accounts, to be a basic part of smart dieting practices. Shouse and Nilsson (2011) assessed the connection between disarranged eating, Intuitive Eating, and self-hushing and found that Intuitive Eating is amplified when a lady has elevated levels of enthusiastic mindfulness, joined with low degrees of self-quieting. Nonetheless, when high passionate mindfulness was combined with increasingly self-quieting, members had progressively confused eating and less Intuitive Eating. The scientists accept that when ladies have clearness about their musings and sentiments, yet quietness their voices, hunger signs may get befuddled, which may diminish trust of inward signals of craving and satiation. The most intuitive and least disarranged eaters in the examination showed high passionate mindfulness and low self-quieting. The aftereffects of this investigation approve the standards: Challenge the Food Police and Cope with Your Emotions without Using Food.

ACKNOWLEDGMENT AND BODY APPRECIATION

While the capacity to eat intuitively is innate, the probability of staying an Intuitive Eater is affected by the earth, which incorporates family, companions, and culture. Intuitive Eating can be obstructed by a situation that needs acknowledgment as well as forces inflexible standards for eating that disregard an individual's internal encounter, (for example, appetite or fulfillment). Moreover, when individuals urge others to be incredulous of their bodies, they (ladies particularly) figure out how to eat in a separated way trying to control their appearance, rather than tuning in to their bodies. Also, strain to get in shape by relatives, companions, and culture (in lieu of body acknowledgment) adds to concentrating on appearance-related eating. Numerous individuals are shocked to discover that body praises can be a type of making a decision about an individual by their appearance, for example, "You look extraordinary—how much weight did you lose?" or "I wish I had a body like yours."

ACCEPTANCE MODEL OF INTUITIVE EATING

A progression of concentrates by Tracy Tylka and associates (Avalos and Tylka 2006, Augustus-Horvath and Tylka 2011), on almost 600 school ladies and 800 ladies ages eighteen to sixty-five years of age, individually, found that putting accentuation on body capacity and body thankfulness are key approaches to make an interpretation of body acknowledgment into Intuitive Eating practices. At the point when ladies stress the usefulness of their bodies over appearance, they are increasingly disposed to eat as indicated by their body's organic prompts. Besides, they found that receiving a mentality of body gratefulness anticipated Intuitive Eating, in light of the fact that good body frames of mind are related with more prominent attention to body signals, joined with a more noteworthy inclination to respect these signs. Their examination demonstrates that it is imperative to advance a positive body direction, which centers on body gratefulness and body usefulness, as opposed to appearance, which thusly, encourages Intuitive Eating.

Tylka and partners found that body gratefulness was remarkably and decidedly identified with Intuitive Eating in a wide assortment of age bunches for ladies. They distinguished four signs of body appreciation:

1. Having a positive assessment of the body in spite of size and saw blemishes.

2. Monitoring and mindful to the body's needs.

3. Taking part in sound practices to deal with the body.

4. Securing the body by dismissing ridiculous media body beliefs.

Tylka and partners accept that it is essential to challenge Western declaration of the meager perfect generalization and advance acknowledgment of an assorted variety of body sizes.

CULTURE ACCEPTANCE

An entrancing arrangement of multi-social investigations by Hawks and associates demonstrate that before and during the beginning times of westernization, people from their local nations are normal Intuitive Eaters, yet this procedure of eating is relinquished to the detriment of the westernized flimsy perfect (Hawks et al. 2004b, Madanat and Hawks 2004).

During cultural assimilation, the westernized standard of excellence becomes disguised, by means of the assault of unreasonable media pictures of slimness, and indigenous Intuitive Eating styles dissolve away, toward outer signals of eating, the two of which can prompt stoutness and eating issue. These acknowledgments examines bolster and approve Principle 7—Respect Your Body.

Shouldn't something be said about Men? A significant number of the Intuitive Eating examines have been directed on ladies or on blended gatherings of people, yet not men as it were. There are considers in progress investigating Intuitive Eating issues in men. A fundamental report on 181 school men by Gast and partners (in press) found that men scoring high on the Hawks' Intuitive Eating Scale were related with a lower weight list, contrasted with men with low Intuitive Eating scores. The men likewise set more an incentive on being physically fit and sound, as opposed to on a perfect weight. The scientists recommended that Intuitive Eating appears to be obviously appropriate for men since it expands on men's enemy of dieting sees (men regularly see dieting practices as ladylike), and expands on self-care wellness convictions that have all the earmarks of being almost certain held by men.

INTUITIVE EATING IS A LIFESTYLE:

Figuring out how to tune in to your body and regard your its astuteness is definitely not a stylish dieting approach like others that have traveled every which way throughout the years. Or maybe, eating intuitively is a methodology that can turn into a natural piece of your life. The ideas are basic yet significantly ground-breaking when put to utilize.

As intuitive eating is training and a lifestyle, as opposed to a pre-set dinner plan that you essentially need to hold fast to, it's not 100 percent precise constantly. A few days you may think that its simple to tune in to your body's internal signals. Different days it might be all the more a battle. Yet, as you work on tuning in, the whole methodology will come all the more effectively and be increasingly reliable after some time. What's more, the advantages as far as self-information, genuine feelings of serenity, and ideal health will be significantly broader than anything you can understand from a common weight reduction diet.

Here, we love educating about eating intuitively. We accept unequivocally that nobody find out about you than YOU. So as you consider all the data out there with respect to food and health make a stride back and look inside. You have such a large amount of the data you need inside your very own body. Your activity is just to work on tuning in.

CONCLUSION

These rules condense the parts of this book. The request where they're introduced isn't a flat out, similarly as nothing in this book is outright, aside from surrendering the quest for dieting. Use them as your formula card, as we recommended toward the starting as far as possible of this book. Be that as it may, similarly as you may extemporize in cooking your dish from the composed formula, be imaginative with these rules. Use what feels directly for you, add to them on the off chance that you like, and dispose of what doesn't fit. The main concern is to confide in your gut—utilize your intuitive abilities to feel great with eating and to discharge yourself from the jail of dieting.

STEP BY STEP GUIDELINES

In case you're somebody who cooks, you'll realize that before you figured out how to cook, simply pulling out a formula card may have made you feel on edge about whether the completed mixture could ever look like any cooked dish you'd at any point before observed. So as to increase a solace level in your kitchen, you most likely expected to see a portion of the essential ideas of cooking. In the event that the formula said "stew," you wouldn't have realized the contrast between bubbling, stewing, or sautéing. The accompanying rules are like your formula card. In the event that you take a gander at them before you read the remainder of the book, you may get confounded and misconstrue the motivation behind each. When you've gotten settled with the Intuitive Eating reasoning, how-ever, these rules can turn into a snappy and simple reference when you have to reconnect with the procedure.

STAGE 1—PRINCIPLE ONE: REJECT THE DIET MENTALITY

Toss out the diet books and magazine articles that offer you bogus any desire for shedding pounds rapidly, effectively, and for all time. Take advantage of the lies that led you to feel disappointed every time another diet stops working and you regain your full weight. In the event that you permit even one little would like to wait that another and better diet may be hiding around the bend, it will keep you from being allowed to rediscover Intuitive Eating.

1. Make a solid duty to quit any pretense of dieting for an amazing remainder. For whatever length of time that you clutch even the smallest idea, guarantee, or expectation that dieting is in your future, you will undermine your capacity to turn into an Intuitive Eater.

2. Toss out the entirety of your calorie counters and old diet books and articles.

3. At the point when companions talk about the most current prevailing fashion diet or you see a TV ad or magazine article on dieting—abstain from getting brought into the fervor that may emerge. Rather, take a full breath and tenderly guarantee yourself that you are focused on another perspective and feeling about food and eating, and that dieting isn't a piece of this new procedure.

4. Ensure your food limits by declining to enable others to mention to you what to eat, when to eat, or the amount to eat. Secure your body limits by declining to enable others to offer remarks about your weight and body. 5. In the event that you notice that you're feeling defiant or starting to eat unwittingly, check in with yourself to check whether regardless you're clutching diet thinking and diet decides that are setting off this response or in case you're being assaulted by any outside limit intruders.

STAGE 2—PRINCIPLE TWO: HONOR YOUR HUNGER

Keep your body organically bolstered with satisfactory vitality and sugars. Else you can trigger a base drive to indulge.

When you arrive right now of inordinate craving, all expectations of moderate, cognizant eating are brief and unessential.

Figuring out how to respect this first natural sign makes way for re-building trust with yourself and food.

1. Start to tune in to the littlest commotion or feeling that shows that you are encountering hunger, for example, a snarling or protesting stomach, a slight migraine, an absence of mental center, crankiness, absence of vitality, and so forth.

2. When you perceive your natural appetite, make an opportunity to eat.

3. In the event that you disregard this most fundamental flag and get over hungry, it will be extremely difficult to recognize what you truly need to eat or when you've had enough. Test with starting to eat at around a "3" or "4" on the "Craving Discovery Scale."

4. In the event that you don't appear to encounter hunger flags over significant stretches of time, you should take a stab at eating each three to four hours. In the end, your body will become acclimated to being nourished normally and will start to give you trustworthy yearning signals.

5. Remember that in the event that you are debilitated or focused on, hunger signs might be blunted. It's critical to sustain your body on those days, as well, regardless of whether you don't feel the appetite.

6. Be readied—make certain to set aside a few minutes for shopping for food, concocting or picking premade food, and for social occasion snacks or even suppers to place in a lunch pack or to convey in the vehicle. Along these lines, you show regard for your body's signs and can accommodate your needs.

STAGE 3—PRINCIPLE THREE: MAKE PEACE WITH FOOD

Call a détente, stop the food battle! Give yourself un-contingent authorization to eat. In the event that you disclose to yourself that you can't or shouldn't have a specific food, it can prompt serious sentiments of hardship that incorporate with wild desires and, regularly, gorging.

At the point when you at last "yield" to your taboo food, eating will be knowledgeable about such power; it for the most part brings about Last Supper overeating, and overpowering blame.

1. Give yourself unrestricted consent to eat whatever you truly like. Make avocado sincerely equal to lettuce and peach pie comparable to a peach.

2. Be careful with giving yourself "pseudo-authorization" by disclosing to yourself that you can eat what you like, however proceeding to hold blameworthy contemplations about your food decisions. It won't work!

3. Try not to deny yourself of any food that sounds engaging you.

4. See how your body feels when eating this food and that it is so fulfilling to your tongue. Give careful consideration of these encounters for your memory bank.

5. Keep a plentiful stockpile of the considerable number of foods that you figure you may get a kick out of the chance to eat. (Restock the sup-employ when it gets low.)

STAGE 4—PRINCIPLE FOUR: CHALLENGE THE FOOD POLICE

Shout a boisterous "NO" to considerations in your mind that pronounce you're "acceptable" for eating negligible calories or "awful" on the grounds that you ate a bit of chocolate cake. The Food Police screen the irrational principles that dieting has made. The police headquarters is housed somewhere down in your mind, and its amplifier yells negative thorns, miserable expressions, and blame inciting arraignments. Pursuing the Food Police away is a basic advance in coming back to Intuitive Eating.

1. Distinguish your mutilated food, dieting, and eating considerations and convictions. Toss them out and supplant them with reality.

2. Tune in for the damaging voices which can talk unsafe considerations:

   a. The Food Police voice is brutal and basic and is driven by the dieting mindset. It very well may be animated by tuning in to the media, guardians, and friends. It keeps you at war with your association with food and your body.

   b. The Nutrition Informant voice is critical and intrigues with the Food Police. It gives you sustenance actualities to help legitimize your dieting.

c. The Diet Rebel voice is irate and is conceived because of limit intruders who traverse the line into the private space that holds your Intuitive Eating signs and emotions about your body. It secures your self-rule while additionally causing some ruinous eating conduct.

3. Build up the accommodating voices that can get you through harsh occasions and make your eating relationship increasingly agreeable:

a. The Food Anthropologist: voice portrays impartial perceptions. It takes note of your considerations and activities as for your food world to assist you with settling on decisions about what you need to eat, when you need to eat, and the amount you have to eat. It can likewise record these musings in your memory bank, so they will be effectively open when required later on to assist you with settling on eating choices.

b. The Nurturer: voice is delicate and delicate and gives calming and consoling articulations that help you through this procedure.

c. The Rebel Ally: voice advances from the Diet Rebel voice and encourages you secure your limits against any individual who attacks your eating space.

d. The Nutrition Ally voice replaces the Nutrition Informant voice when the Food Police are ousted. It is keen on good dieting with no concealed dieting motivation.

The Intuitive Eater voice addresses your gut responses. You were brought into the world with this voice, and it offers you messages and responses about your eating that no one but you can know. It additionally causes you settle on choices that lone you reserve the option to make.

4. Watch out for negative self-talk dependent on the accompanying silly convictions and contorted reasoning:

a. Dichotomous intuition—thinking in a win or bust, high contrast design.

b. Absolutist reasoning—magical thinking that accepts that one conduct will completely influence and control a subsequent conduct.

c. Catastrophic intuition—thinking in misrepresented ways.

d. Pessimistic reasoning — where a given circumstance is found in its most dire outcome imaginable.

e. Linear deduction—thinking in a straight line, taking into consideration no factors, concentrating on the final products.

5. Supplant negative self-chat with positive self-talk dependent on balanced reasoning. A few instances of objective reasoning include:

a. Living in the dim—moderate considerations, not highly contrasting.
b. Permissive considerations and articulations.
c. Accurate, non-overstated considerations.
d. Process thinking—center on consistent change and getting the hang of, organizing the methods as opposed as far as possible.

STAGE 5: PRINCIPLE FIVE: FEEL YOUR PLENITY

Tune the body flags that reveal that you will never be anxious again. Observe the signs indicating that it is easily refillable. Relax during a party or meal and ask yourself how you know the food and what your current level of completion is.

1. Focus on your completion signals. However, recollect, the main way that you can do this is to give yourself unequivocal consent to eat. You should immovably accept that you will have the option to eat again when you get eager so as to have the option to stop when you're full.

2. Make certain to respect your craving. In case you're eager for over, your desperation to eat will make extraordinary trouble in perceiving your completion signals. Similarly, in the event that you start eating before obvious craving emerges, your totality signs will be quieted—you're probably going to be guided by your tongue rather than your stomach.

3. Dispose of the thought that you should complete everything on your plate since you dread squandering food. Unmistakably more harm should be possible to your body and your mind by eating additional food than by disposing of it.

4. Increment your awareness so as to assist you with recognizing satiety.

   a. Try eating without interruption so you can be completely present during your supper.

   b. Pause in a feast or tidbit and take an opportunity to check your completion level. This isn't a pledge to quit eating yet a promise to check in with your body and taste buds.

Take a taste check. Ask, "How does the food taste? Does it live up to your desires? Is it fulfilling your taste buds? Or on the other hand would you say you are proceeding to eat in light of the fact that it's there?"

Take a satiety check. Focus on the signs that your stomach offers you to demonstrate that you're turning out to be comfortably full. Ask, "What's my appetite or completion level? Am I still eager? Is hunger leaving? Do I feel voracious? Am I starting to feel fulfilled?"

   c. Identify the Last Bite Threshold. This is the endpoint. You realize that the nibble of food in your mouth is the last. Try not to stress on the off chance that you can't do this from the start—it will at last become intuitive. On the off chance that you feel disillusioned that you need to stop now, recollect, you can eat this food or food once more, when your appetite returns.

Eating is in reality all the more fulfilling when you're serenely eager, as opposed to effectively full. You're giving yourself a blessing by halting at this point.

d. Make a solid explanation to yourself that you've arrived at the limit chomp by putting your fork and blade on your plate or by pushing your plate ahead a smidgen.

e. Give your remains to the server to wrap up in case you're at a café or placed them in the fridge in case you're at home.

f. Say, "No, thank you" immovably to your host or entertainer if more food is being pushed onto you. You reserve an option to state "no."

5. Ensure that you have a lot of food profit capable for your suppers. In the event that you give yourself too little to even think about eating, you'll never feel fulfilled or full. You don't require "to an extreme" food, yet "excessively little" food will attack this procedure.

6. Select foods that have some substance. On the off chance that you just pick "air foods, for example, rice cakes and crude vegetables, you'll get a misguided feeling of satiety, just to get eager again far and away too rapidly. Feed yourself "genuine food."

STAGE 6—PRINCIPLE SIX: DISCOVER THE SATISFACTION FACTOR

The Japanese have the intelligence to advance delight as one of their objectives of sound living. In our rage to be meager and solid, we frequently disregard one of the most fundamental blessings of presence—the joy and fulfillment that can be found in the eating experience. When you eat what you really need, in a welcoming and favorable situation, the joy you bring will be an incredible power to help you feel satisfied and satisfied. By giving this experience to yourself, you will find that it takes significantly less food to choose you've had "enough."

1. Give yourself authorization to look for delight in your eating. The more pleasurable your food is, the more fulfillments you'll get from your eating experience. (The more fulfilled you feel, the less you'll have to eat—particularly on the off chance that you realize that this food will never be illegal.)

2. Make sense of what you truly need to eat by focusing on the accompanying sensations related with eating:

   a. Taste—sweet, appetizing, salty, acrid, or unpleasant
   b. Surface—hard, crunchy, smooth, rich, and so forth.
   c. Smell—sweet, harsh, gentle, and so forth.
   d. Appearance—shading, shape, eye claim, and so forth.
   e. Temperature—hot, cool, cold, calm
   f. Volume or filling limit—vaporous, light, thick

3. Consider how your body may feel when you complete the process of eating:

    a. Will you be physically fulfilled by your decision?

    b. Will thick food make you feel awkwardly full later or a breezy food leaves you feeling unfilled?

    c. Will an excessively rich supper give you stomach trouble?

    d. Will an essentially sweet dinner send your glucose on an exciting ride?

4. Make your eating condition charming:

    a. Eat when delicately hungry as opposed to eager for over.

    b. Make time to value your food.

    c. Create a stylish domain—attempt pretty placemats, candles, vivid dishes, traditional music. Keep the clamor level down.

    d. Sit down to eat.

    e. Take a few full breaths before you eat.

    f. Savor your food.

    g. Pay consideration regarding eating as gradually as possible.

    h. Taste each nibble of food that you put in your mouth.

    i. Provide assortment in your supper.

    j. Avoid pressure while eating.

5. Try not to settle. Wipe out the unenjoyable—in the event that you don't cherish it, don't eat it, and on the off chance that you love it, relish it!

6. Check in with your taste buds amidst your dinner to check whether the food still tastes in the same class as it did when you started.

7. Keep in mind; it doesn't generally need to be great—a few times suppers are not in your control. There are a lot more open doors ahead for fulfilling suppers.

STAGE 7-PRINCIPLE SEVEN: COPE WITH YOUR EMOTIONS WITHOUT USING FOOD

Discover approaches to comfort, sustain, divert, and resolve your issues without utilizing food. Nervousness, depression, weariness, and outrage are feelings we as a whole encounter all through life. Everyone has its very own trigger, and every ha its very own submission. Food won't fix any of these sentiments. It might comfort for the present moment, divert from the torment, or even numb you into a food headache; however food won't take care of the issue. In the event that anything, eating for an enthusiastic yearning will just exacerbate you feel over the long haul. You'll eventually need to manage the wellspring of the feeling, just as the distress of overeating.

1. Ask yourself: "Am I organically eager?" If your answer is truly, respect your appetite and eat!

2. When you end up looking for food however realize that you're not organically eager, take an opportunity to ask yourself, "What am I feeling?"

   a. Are you frightened, restless, furious, exhausted, harmed, desolate, discouraged? Or then again would you say you are upbeat, energized, need a prize, or need to celebrate?

   b. To help recognize your sentiments, invest some tranquil energy writing in your diary or talking into a recording device. Or on the other hand, if it's simpler to connect with your sentiments with someone else, call a decent companion or getting relative. You may even need to call your psychotherapist or food specialist. Use email if that is a simpler method to impart.

3. At that point ask yourself, "What do I need?"

a. Do you really require a rest, an embrace, some intelligent incitement, and so on.? Food doesn't properly fulfill any of those requirements.

4. So as to get your needs met, ask: "Would you please?" Sometimes, for should be satisfied, you'll need to make some noise and request help.

5. Address your issues without utilizing food in the accompanying manners:

a. Nurture yourself by washing up, tuning in to relieving music, getting a back rub, taking a yoga class, getting yourself a few blooms, and so on.

b. Deal with your emotions. Recognize what is disturbing you. Enable your sentiments to develop. This will diminish your need to drive them down with food.

c. If vital, give yourself an impermanent interruption. It's alright to escape from the sentiments now and again, yet you don't need to utilize food for this reason. Have a go at leasing a motion picture, perusing an engrossing book, tuning in to music or a book recording, cultivating, and so forth.

6. On the off chance that you have a scene of utilizing food to adapt, consider it to be a warning that something is going on in your life that requirements consideration. Whatever you do, don't pound yourself for this conduct. The vast majorities do it now and again—simply accept it as a learning encounter and go on.

STAGE 8—PRINCIPLE EIGHT: RESPECT YOUR BODY

Acknowledge your hereditary outline. Similarly as an individual with a shoe size of eight would not hope to sensibly press into a size six, it is similarly as worthless (and awkward) to have a similar desire with body size. In any case, for the most part, regard your body, so you can rest easy thinking about who you are. It's difficult to dismiss the diet attitude in the event that you are unreasonable and excessively basic about your body shape.

1. Value the pieces of your body that you particularly like—regardless of whether it's your hair, midriff, feet, or nose.

2. Scrub down, and use salves and creams that vibe calming as you focus on them.

3. Get back rubs and embraces and strokes that offer your body the chance to be contacted.

4. Get settled. Purchase agreeable under-articles of clothing. Purchase apparel that is complimenting and fits you without being tight.

5. Try not to conceal your body in garments that are excessively huge.

6. Stop the body-check game. Quit contrasting yourself with every other person in the room. It blinds you from valuing yourself and is an arrangement for more body disappointment. It may even make a compulsion to come back to dieting.

7. Try not to bargain for the "Huge Event." Don't capitulate to the weight of "dieting down" to press into that uncommon outfit—it wills just blowback.

8. Stop body slamming. Each time you center on your defective body parts, it makes progressively hesitance and body stress. At the point when you hear yourself offering deriding remarks about your body, supplant these remarks with kind body proclamations.

9. Quit gauging yourself. It can just make you feel disappointed with your body.

10. Regard body decent variety, particularly yours.

11. Be reasonable about your hereditary cosmetics. Acknowledge your body type, and realize that your body is probably going to adjust at its regular weight when you're reliably tuning in to your intuitive signals and rehearsing self-care.

12. Be comprehension of yourself. Regard the way that you might be higher than your ordinary body weight on the off chance that you are somebody who has utilized food to adapt

when you realized no other method to deal with your emotions, or in light of the fact that you've been a casualty of the diet attitude. Be delicate with yourself and acknowledge that your body is the place it is on the grounds that you had next to no decision about these variables.

STAGE 9—PRINCIPLE NINE: EXERCISE—FEEL THE DIFFERENCE

Disregard aggressor work out. Simply get dynamic and feel the distinction. Shift your focus on how it feels to move your body, as opposed to the impact of calorie-consuming activity. On the off chance that you center on how you feel from turning out, for example, empowered, it can have the effect between turning up for an energetic morning walk and hitting the rest alarm. On the off chance that when you wake up, your solitary objective is to get more fit, it's typically not an inspiring element at that time of time.

1. Leap forward exercise obstructions:

   a. Discover every one of the purposes for any activity obstruction that you may have. It might be expected to having been prodded as a kid, having re-belled against power, feeling threatened for not having a fit enough body, and so forth.

   b. Focus on how it feels. Exercise is basically for feeling better. It so happens that the better you feel, the less you'll have to utilize food as an approach to adapt. It can likewise give you expanded vitality, a general atmosphere of prosperity, a feeling of strengthening, and sounder rest.

    c. Disassociate practice from weight reduction. Delete the tape of how exercise felt when you were dieting. You presumably weren't getting enough calories or starches to give you the vitality to exercise and feel great simultaneously.

    d. Focus on practice as a method for dealing with yourself, feeling great now and forestalling medical issues further down the road.

    e. Don't get trapped in practice mind games, for example,

    f. The, It's-Not-Worth It Trap—i.e., feeling it's not justified, despite any potential benefits in the event that it doesn't last a predetermined measure of time.

    g. Couch-Potato Denial—being occupied isn't equivalent to physical action.

    h. The No-Time-to-Spare Trap—figures out how to prioritize.

    i. The If-I-Don't-Sweat-It-Doesn't-Count Trap—physical wellness doesn't need to mean thorough exercises.

2. Get dynamic in day by day living. Make practice helpful and fun:

    a. Park your vehicle a couple of squares from your goal so you can add some strolling to your day.

    b. Walk up stairs as opposed to utilizing the lift.

    c. Ride your bicycle or stroll to work on the off chance that you live close enough.

d. When you travel, take strolling shoes or a bounce rope. Consider picking lodgings that have exercise offices.

3. Make practice fun.

a. Consider playing a group activity, for example, volleyball (sea shore volleyball throughout the late spring), softball, ball, soccer, or tennis.

b. Join an exercise center, if having others around you will propel you.

c. Buy a treadmill or other home gym equipment and put a TV and DVR or DVD player before it so you can record and watch motion pictures or fascinating projects. Tuning in to music or a book recording may likewise make the activity progressively fun.

d. Find an activity band together with whom you can go for strolls. Talking and strolling can make the walk progressively charming.

4. Make practice a nonnegotiable need.

5. Be agreeable while working out.

6. Incorporate quality preparing so you can remake muscle that was lost from dieting.

7. Incorporate extending as a feature of your activity schedule.

8. Remember rest. Ensure you give yourself long stretches of rest inside your activity week. It will forestall burnout, just as allowing your muscles to invigorate and fix.

STAGE 10: TEN PRINCIPLE: HONOR YOUR HEALTH WITH SOFT NUTRITION

Decide on food decisions that respect your health and taste buds while making you feel good. Remember that it is not necessary to follow an ideal diet to be solid. Suddenly, you will not miss a supplement or get fat for a bite, a party or a day of food. It's what you eat reliably after some time that issues. Progress, not flawlessness, is what matters.

1. Think about the precepts of food insight: assortment, control, and equalization. Likewise with work out, think about food as your identification into feeling better.

2. Feed your digestion. Make certain to stir your metabolic fire by getting adequate fuel for the duration of the day by eating at whatever point you're eager.

3. Eat a lot of entire grains, leafy foods, and beans for their fiber content, so your stomach related tract functions admirably. They're likewise a force place of nutrients, minerals, and phyto-synthetics.

4. Eat adequate protein, yet not all that much, for cell fix and creation of hormones, compounds, hair, nails, and so forth.

5. Eat a lot of starches and adequate calories so your protein can be utilized as a protein source and not be signed as a vitality source.

6. Take in a sufficient measure of dairy items to get enough calcium to keep your bones solid.

7. Drink a lot of water to help processing, forestall stoppage, have adequate blood volume, and wash down your kidneys.

8. Eat a sufficient measure of fat. We need fat in our diets consequently:

   a. to advance satiety,
   b. to help manufacture cell dividers, including synapses,
   c. for retention of fat solvent nutrients, and
   d. for creation of hormones.
   e. Whenever conceivable, pick quality fats, for example, avocado, olive oil, nuts, and so forth.

9. Take into account some play foods so as to offset your great health with joy and fulfillment. Leave the vast majority of your food decisions alone made for physical health, while some of them are for basic delight.

10. Try not to be tricked by the fat-free trip. Fat free doesn't mean calorie free or supplement thick. These foods will in general be restricted in supplements, while having an excess of sugar. Without fat foods frequently are not as fulfilling as low-fat foods. They likewise make a fantasy of being low-calorie and lead to overconsumption before you know it.

11. Get off the food pedestal. You don't need to be great. Respect your health, your taste buds, and your humanness.

CPSIA information can be obtained
at www.ICGtesting.com
Printed in the USA
BVHW041041201120
593711BV00022B/173